Other Books by the Author:

Dr. Cantor's Longevity Diet

UNITROL: The Healing Magic of the Mind

Alpha-Theta UNITROL: How to Turn On the Power of the Mind

Doctor Cantor's Secrets of Self-Revitalization

Alfred J. Cantor, M.D.

Parker Publishing Company, Inc.
West Nyack, New York

This book is a reference work based on research by the author. The opinions expressed herein are not necessarily those of or endorsed by the publisher. The directions stated in this book are in no way to be considered as a substitute for consultation with a duly licensed doctor.

Library of Congress Cataloging in Publication Data

Cantor, Alfred Joseph
Doctor Cantor's Secrets of self-revitalization.

Includes index.
1. Health. 2. Vitality. 3. Diet.
4. Holistic medicine. I. Title. II. Title:
Secrets of self-revitalization.
RA776.5.C33 613 79-9525
ISBN 0-13-216382-9

Printed in the United States of America

For—Eleanor, Pam, Lauren, Jeffrey and Alfred Jay
With all my love

My special gratitude, as always, goes with my eternal love, to Eleanor, Pam and Jay, for their constant, unfailing encouragement during difficult times.

To Lauren, I offer a kiss and a hug, and the hope that she will remember "Poppy" and his "magic" with love.

My work was prepared under the auspices of the Unitrol Institute for Research in Geriatrics, Inc.

To all my patients and students of UNITROL, I hope this book will bring still more happiness, pleasure, comfort and renewed vitality—long life and joy in each day.

FOREWORD

Dr. Cantor is one of those rare physicians who takes nothing for granted, but researches his subject with meticulous care and thoroughness. Because of this, he is able to write for the medical practitioner as though the doctor were a layman and for the layman as though he or she were a physician. Anyone can readily understand the concepts presented so simply and with unusual clarity in his writings. Reading over the books he has written, we see a medical mind of the first order at work, to whom the health and well-being of others is a vital concern.

The questions he tackles are basic ones. For example—"What is illness?" and "When is a person 'sick'?" There is an ancient Eastern tale which states that, in China, the doctor gets paid only when his patient is *well.* This seems to be Cantor's motto. He is concerned with how each person can become revitalized and rejuvenated. In his discussion, he clarifies mind-body relationships, problems of nutrition and the various methods of relaxation among many other things, and his approach seems as valid when disease is not yet present as when the person is bedridden or otherwise immobilized.

Those of us interested in treating the *whole person* recognize that medical responsibility begins long before disease appears, and at this time in medical development, this approach is increasingly of the essence. It is modern in an honest sense, and it bears significantly on what the professional refers to as "holistic medicine."

In this book, Dr. Cantor updates his remarkably researched and clinically proven concepts of restoring and maintaining health and vitality, and the topics he covers are of universal importance. Can life be prolonged? Can youthful aliveness be regained? Can a greater sprightliness and meaningfulness of mental and bodily functioning be recaptured? Can hope and a sense of joy be awakened in human beings who have precipitately decided, "Oh, what's the use? It's all over. Nothing lies ahead." Dr. Cantor's clarion call—his enthusiastic faith in the holistic perspective—evokes the excitement of better things to come. People can and *do* live longer now, and the aging process *can* be combatted successfully.

Taking nothing for granted, Dr. Cantor's program is practical and his holistic approach is presented in a detailed program that the reader can readily follow. It is a "no nonsense" statement which can be useful in endless ways to the laity and professionals alike. He cautions, however, that the advice of a personal physician is essential in many instances, especially if the reader's problem involves such complicated pathology as cancer or other diseases of like nature. And after the recognized treatments, such as surgery, radiation and/or chemotherapy, and if the oncologist approves, the revitalization program described by the author can be used to stimulate the immune system, strengthen the cells and tissues of the organs, and assist the "body-mind" in delaying or even "curing" the further spread of such illnesses.

This is truly the New Medicine! To "keep in touch," professionals nowadays not only proclaim the revitalizing rewards of the new holistic benefits of modern ways in medicine—as an ever growing area of well attended medical and scientific conferences proves—but they also practice these guidelines in their own lives.

What is particularly impressive in Dr. Cantor's book is that the author speaks from the vantage point of forty years of experience, not only as a nutritionist, but also as a distinguished surgeon. He was among the first to recognize the importance of early ambulation after surgery, which will earn him a permanent place in medicine. His textbook, "Early Ambulation," has no doubt saved many lives in all parts of the world. Beaumont S. Cornell, M.D., the distinguished Editor-in-Chief of an eminent gastroenterology journal, pointed out the importance of Dr. Cantor's contribution in the introduction to that landmark book almost forty years ago!

Many people who are eating more fish today than ever before, who are drinking bottled hard water, who are limiting their food to half-portions and who are practicing body-mind techniques such as meditation, Yoga, Zen and the like, may first have learned about these concepts directly or indirectly from the author's books on "Unitrol" and the "Longevity Diet."

They may possibly have taken advice from his very early books on psychosomatic medicine, written originally for the physician. Lay people may know of his total body-mind, holistic approach from his popular books such as "Ridding Yourself of Psychosomatic Health Wreckers," "How to Lose Weight the Doctor's Way," "Immortality—Pathways to Peace of Mind" and "Cancer Can be Cured" (the latter has been published in many languages).

In a large way, the author is a "healer" in the true medical sense of the word. His objective is to teach how to "heal" oneself, yet always with the caution that one should work closely with one's physician when necessary. I have always been impressed by Dr. Cantor's genuine gift for understanding the essential human being in terms of the richness of his or her potential for happiness and fullness of living—and my opinion is amply justified by the present book.

Harmon S. Ephron, M.D.
Clinical Professor, Dept. of Psychiatry
Rutgers Medical College
Piscataway, N.J.

INTRODUCTION

The purpose of this book is to offer 17 lengthy consultations, as if you were a patient in my offices, each consultation designed to show you how to revitalize your body. You will learn how to strengthen your body-mind, restore energy where necessary, restore youth where possible, prolong life in many cases, and I will also show you how to enjoy a healthier, more vital lifestyle and regain joy in living.

If you were to pay for these consultations they would cost you over a thousand dollars. Through the magic of printing and publishing, you receive all this information, all these consultations and can refer to them again and again—as if you were returning to my offices each time—for a very tiny fraction of that amount.

Let me begin by explaining to you that each of us is unique. Just as there are no two people with the same fingerprints, there are no two people with the same cell structure, the same tissue structure, the same organ structure or the same body-mind. Each of us is totally unique in every respect. The general pattern appears to be the same, but again—just like fingerprints—it is not the same.

The next principle I wish to explain is that each disease has multiple causes. These causes may be generally classified as genetic (the type of tissue you are born with), your internal and external environment (the thoughts that have been programmed in your mind and the physical environment both outside and within your body as your cells, tissues and organs function) and your nutrition. These are the three most important factors that determine whether or not your tissues have sufficient vitality to live through the next heartbeat, the next minute, the next hour, the next day—indeed, they determine how many years you will live and the state of your health during that time. Your health varies from moment to moment, day to day. We all go through cycles in many ways. You can see this most clearly in the female menstrual cycle. But there are many other cycles; some within the body itself, some in our environment and all interacting to cause variations in your health from moment to moment. This variation in vitality once again makes you unique, since your variations will be different from those of any other person.

If you are aging prematurely and lack energy and vitality, your entire body-mind must be reevaluated and revitalized. In this book I will teach you the meaning of "food for the mind." I will teach you how to empty your mind of self-destructive programmed thinking, self-destructive thought patterns and fixed ideas. I will show you that stress, although necessary to some degree, can kill if excessive.

I will also teach you how to attain the silent mind. It is only the silent mind, emptied of fixed patterns of the past, that can develop new, creative patterns in the present and the future. Now to the question of food for the body. Please note that although I use these terms, I never think of the body alone. It is always a body-mind. We will not be dealing with the government nutritional requirements called MDR (minimal daily requirements), because this equals minimal daily vitality.

We will not be dealing with RDA (recommended daily allowances), for this offers only a slightly better daily vitality than minimal daily requirements. We will be dealing in our consultations with ODR (optimal daily requirements).

Optimal daily requirements must be made to order, since we are each unique. Of course, there are general rules that are applicable for most of us, otherwise I could not be writing a book for the general public.

Poorly functioning cells, tissues and organs require special nutrients, sometimes in large dosage. I must caution you to see your doctor first if you are not feeling well. Request a complete physical, chemical and emotional study. If your doctor is not particularly interested in or knowledgeable about nutrition, take a copy of your diagnostic studies to a nutritionist and to any other specialist he may recommend in addition.

Then, try The ODR Revitalization Program. This program, as you will learn when you read the consultations, offers a practical, tested mind-body study that you can put to work immediately. Each consultation is part of the ODR Revitalization Program, the optimal mind-body approach.

You will learn how to empty your mind and be born anew each day.

You will learn how to empty your body of ITPs (internally produced toxic products).

You will learn how to reduce exposure to ETPs (external toxic products).

You will learn how to use nutritional ODR (optimal daily requirements)

- to restore normal cell, tissue and organ functions
- to attain optimal tissue vitality
- to prevent disease
- to strengthen your "immune" system

I would like to tell you something now about the immune system so that you will understand one of the basic concepts upon which my consultations are founded. It is generally accepted theory that a certain number of cancer cells are produced in each person each day. Obviously, we would all die of cancer very quickly if we did not have a natural immune mechanism to control and/or destroy such cells.

It is important to recognize that the nutrition of each individual cell is basic in the functioning of this immune system. If the nutrition is not optimal, the functioning will not be optimal, and cancer may very well develop to the point of total destruction of the organism. The nutrition of each individual cell is also basic to the activation of lymphocyte production. There are certain lymphocytes (white blood cells of a special defense force) that are apparently most important in warding off or reversing cancer cell formation.

We also have important information to indicate that a particular vitamin we will discuss in detail later is most important in the production of the intercellular material called "collagen," that holds our tissues together. This same vitamin is of basic importance to the function of the very important glands that lie on top of each kidney (the adrenal glands).

Obviously, there are other still unknown elements in the immune system, not yet sufficiently researched for publication, that must be revitalized if the *total* immune system is to function adequately in the control and revitalization of body functions and prevention of disease—even cancer. It is my theory that only by providing the optimal daily requirements (ODR) of both known and unknown nutrients and by avoiding (where possible) the destructive internal and external toxic products can we strengthen and reinforce our immune system.

This is what I call holistic medicine—understanding and treating the entire body-mind and its external and internal environment. This is what I mean by revitalization.

Alfred J. Cantor, M.D.

A Tribute to All Physicians, Authors, Lecturers and Researchers.

During the past forty-seven years, since my medical school days, I have been privileged to study the literature of many countries, in medical books, journals and published papers, as well as in the lecture halls and in correspondence with researchers in the United States and abroad.

This literature has covered the most recent information on nutrition, the recently recognized relationship between nutrition and cancer, and indeed the entire gamut of medicine as it relates to the health of mind and body.

Since a bibliography to recount the list of the total range of publications would require a book many times the size of the one you now hold in your hand, I can only speak with gratitude for the many contributions that have been made by my colleagues in the profession.

A free and generous exchange of information in the medical profession is and should be a source of pride for all physicians. The research continues, now with even greater emphasis on the relationship between nutrition and many diseases, including cardiovascular problems and malignancy of all parts of the body, *the two major causes of premature aging and death.*

To be fully updated, always consult your personal physician, and follow his instructions.

Contents

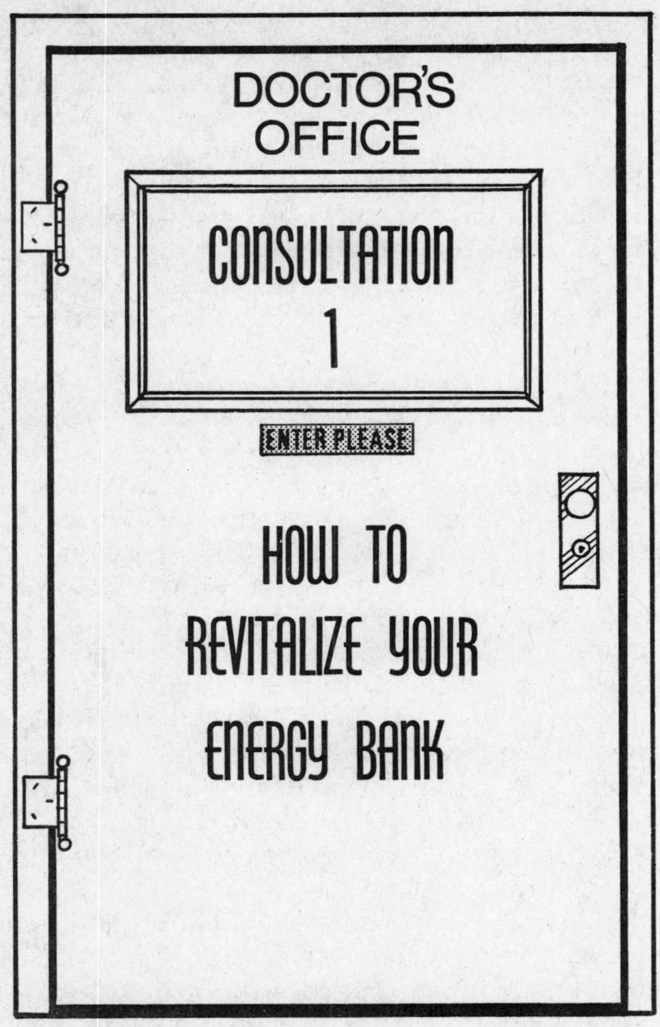

DOCTOR'S
OFFICE
CONSULTATION
1
ENTER PLEASE
HOW TO
REVITALIZE YOUR
ENERGY BANK

By Way of Introduction

You and I are now comfortably seated in my consultation room, and I should like to tell you something about your "energy bank" before we begin this consultation.

What do I mean by "energy bank"? Each of your body's cells is a complete energy unit, and the entire body is made up of such cells. The cells function in cooperation with all other cells and organs in your body. To function properly, they require many chemicals and oxygen; the chemicals coming from your food and water and the oxygen coming from the air you breathe. Without a full, complete, optimal level of nutrients, water and oxygen, your energy bank (total cell-organs) will not maintain your body in the best of health.

Most of us do not have optimal levels of food, pure water and air, and many of us are exposed to toxic chemicals in the water we drink, the food we eat and the air we breathe. The result is a depletion of our energy banks at the cellular, organ and total body levels.

In this book, in each of our consultations, I hope to fully inform and instruct you so that you will know how to provide the best possible levels and combinations of energy-producing foods, water and air to your system in order to revitalize and restore your personal energy bank to the most effective functional levels. When you do this, you will be revitalizing, perhaps even rejuvenating, your body. You may well be prolonging your life at the same time that you restore your youth and vitality.

Think of this program as recharging your "battery." Indeed, each cell is a tiny chemical "battery" with incredibly complex molecules. If you do not feed your cells with optimal levels of nutrients, they will age prematurely and die. I hope to teach you all that you need to know so that you will reverse the aging process and restore better health and new youth to every cell in your body—recharging your energy banks every minute of the day and night.

And now, let me introduce myself. I am a graduate of the College of Medicine of Syracuse University and have been practicing medicine and surgery for the past forty years. I have written fourteen published books, the first being a surgical textbook on a specialty that I created, ambulatory proctology. My concept was that the patient who walked off the operating table approximately one-half hour after surgery, went home to recuperate and returned the next day to the office, would have fewer complications and be back at work much more rapidly than the patient who is kept at rest in a hospital bed for one or two weeks. The concept of early or immediate ambulation is now generally accepted and has probably saved millions of lives during the past forty years.

The next book that I wrote dealt with the psychosomatic aspects of intestinal disorders. In this book, I indicated that all disease is psychosomatic, even cancer, in the sense that there is always an emotional as well as a physical component—at the very least—in each disease. It is therefore necessary to treat the whole person and it is not enough to simply prescribe a drug or advise an operation.

You may have read some of my work on longevity, dealing with health in terms of diet and nutrition, or on Unitrol, discussing health in terms of methods to control the health of the mind as well as the body. I believe in holistic medicine. This involves the treatment of the entire patient as a single unit, a mind-body in an environment, and not simply the treatment of the disease, whether it be the common cold, hemorrhoids, premature aging or even cancer. *There are multiple causes for all diseases,* and the true physician should be prepared to treat the entire person as a body-mind—a living, breathing, feeling, anxiety-ridden human being. With this brief introduction, I believe that you now know a little bit about my background, who I am and what I stand for.

Truth Is Change

We cannot step in the same stream twice. The stream of knowledge, like any stream of water, is constantly flowing, constantly changing. That which is true today may not be true tomorrow. Certainly, yesterday's truths are for the most part today's history of man's attempt to find answers, but are not necessarily today's truths. Therefore, "truth is change."

You must keep an open mind, a practically "emptied" mind, if you are ever to achieve truth. And when you have reached a conclusion that you believe to be "true," be prepared at all times to accept a new "truth" that is closer to reality than the one on which you have based your thinking up to that time.

A Few Words of Caution

And so, I come now to a few words of caution. First, do not depend upon books, not my book or any other book, if you are ill, aging more rapidly than you should or for any reason feel the need to restore your energy. See your doctor first. Have him study your problem completely and carefully, and then follow his advice in every way.

Each of us is unique. Your capacity for each function of your body is totally different from that of any other living person or anyone who has ever lived before. Your genetic structure—the tissues with which you are born—is determined at the time of conception and depends upon which sperm meets which egg. Since each sperm carries a different coded message and each egg is also totally unique, the individual that results is different from all others who have ever lived before or who will ever live in the future. It is like the patterns of snowflakes or fingerprints; all different, never once repeated.

Therefore, you must be studied as a unique individual, and your doctor must advise you on the basis of your own personal, totally individual needs. If he disagrees with anything I say, have said or will say in this book, or in any of my other books, do as your doctor tells you. I can only talk about my own experience, my personal life, the patients I have treated, the problems I have been consulted for, but your special needs can only be determined by a careful examination by your personal physician and any other consultants he may require.

And now, another word of caution. My studies of the literature in medicine and my evaluations of that literature, as well as the experience of forty years in the practice of medicine, have led me to certain general conclusions as to how the body functions and how it loses its capacity to prevent aging and restore youth. What I have done in these consultations is to give you certain general observations regarding these functions. I believe that my suggestions will be helpful for many, hopefully for you. My objective is to show you how to slow aging and restore vitality to aging cells, tissues and organs. But the process may have gone too far; you will need the help of your personal physician in making that determination.

And now, for a final word of caution. We cannot all tolerate or benefit from the same diet, the same level of protein, carbohydrate or fat, the same amounts of vitamins or minerals. Indeed, there are many unknown elements yet to be discovered in our food and even in the water that we drink and the air that we breathe.

As a simple example, if you are overweight and another reader of these consultations is underweight, you will obviously require different approaches to diet. If you lack certain vitamins or certain minerals, you will obviously need a larger supply of these than you have been taking in your food, perhaps even more than those required as the minimal daily requirements for the average person.

Since there is no such thing as an "average person," good judgment must be used in reaching the final decision. I will advise you only on what I consider to be the optimal daily requirements of food and water and the optimal daily requirements of vitamins and minerals. But, even these amounts cannot be considered fixed for all time and for all people. Remembering that we are each unique in every way, you should seek the advice of your personal physician in making a final evaluation.

In my opinion, you can restore much vitality to your energy bank. Unless you are presently suffering from a terminal illness, you can bring about many changes in your energy levels. During these consultations, I will do my best to teach you what I have learned about such changes during the past forty years of medical practice.

I will also tell you the basic approaches you can use to provide not only the best food for your body, but the best food for your mind as well. These opinions will be based on the conclusions of a total lifetime of study and the practice of the teachings of Eastern religions and Western thought.

††*The Strange Case of Dr. A.*

Dr. A. is my closest friend. He has lived an exemplary life as it relates to nutrition. He has never smoked, rarely takes coffee or tea, eats a half-portion diet, watches his weight closely and has even written a book on cancer.

I expected Dr. A. to live to be at least one hundred years old, and I was astonished to learn, one day, that he was entering the hospital for surgery. Somehow, he had developed a cancer of the lung. Cancer of the lung, in men, is usually fatal within the first six months after surgery, or surgery and radiation, or chemotherapy. Only seven percent, according to the statistics of the Sloan-Kettering Institute in New York, survive for as long as five years, so the outlook was not good.

How was it that Dr. A., a non-smoker, had developed cancer of the lung? The answer proved to be relatively simple. His consultation room was an enclosed, sound-proof room, with a four-inch thick door between him and his secretary and nurse, who sat just outside the door at their desks. The windows in his consultation room could not be opened. There was no ventilation. Regrettably, he was too gentle to reprimand his nurse and secretary for their habit of smoking. Indeed, every time he even suggested to them that such smoking could cause cancer of the lung, emphysema or other diseases, it seemed that they smoked even more. From packages of cigarettes on the desk, there soon appeared cartons of cigarettes. It was that cigarette smoke, seeping underneath the door to the consultation room, that converted the consultation room into a smoke-filled chamber, with the doctor as the unconscious "target" of the smoke.

Surgery was still possible if his cancer had not spread beyond the lung. Dr. A. subjected himself to the various X-ray studies, scans, and so forth, which are required before entering the hospital for surgery. The scans proved negative; there was no discernable spread of his disease to the bones, the liver, the kidneys, the brain or other organs. Three and one-half years before this writing, he was on the operating table for five or six hours while biopsies were taken from the area between the lungs—the mediastinum—in which lie the great blood vessels and the heart. Fortunately, these biopsies showed no evidence of cancer, and it was possible to proceed with the removal of the middle lobe of the right lung containing the cancer.

When the doctor returned from the hospital, he promptly closed his office, gave up his practice and began an intensive study of the literature on cancer; not only did he study cancer of the lung, but he investigated all types of cancer and read about immunology. Immunology deals with the capacity of the body to provide substances within the bloodstream to reach the cells and fight against all diseases, including cancer.

He learned that in Germany, certain doctors were using a form of vitamin A in conjunction with chemotherapy and extensive radiation in the treatment of cancer with good results. However, that product could not be imported into the United States.

He also learned that in Scotland, Ewan Cameron, M.D. and Dr. Linus Pauling had treated a large number of cancer patients (with cancer in all parts of the body in terminal stages) with vitamin C, the orange juice vitamin. The terminally ill cancer patients treated with large doses of vitamin C lived an average of three or four times as long as those who had no such treatment, were in better health during this extended duration of time and did not die a slow, lingering death when death finally came. Death came abruptly, which is all the better.

At the time of this writing, he learned that a Dr. Michael B. Sporn of the National Cancer Institute in the United States was working with a synthetic form of retinoids, a relative of vitamin A. This substance is called 13-*cis*-retinoic acid. Dr. Sporn has advised the public that vitamin A in its natural form cannot help the cancer process and may be toxic if the dose is very high. But the retinoids (in vitamin A) are not toxic in proper dosage and are essential to normal growth of cells in the lung, the pancreas, the colon, the breast, the bladder and the prostate. If the retinoids or their analogs are found to be effective in blocking the development of cancer in these organs, they will prevent about half of all cancer deaths.

Since studies on animals have shown that the retinoid analog compound will block such malignancy, a test is now being developed to determine whether or not it will do the same for people.

Dr. A. immediately placed himself on a very high-level dosage of vitamin A, since he could not import into this country the preparation being used in Germany. He recognized that he was not using 13-*cis*-retinoic acid, but until it became available, he would take his chances. He took 35,000 units of vitamin A, a very large dosage by ordinary standards and one that might be toxic for some people.

He also took 10 or 12 grams of vitamin C daily, dividing it in such fashion that he takes one-third of the dose after breakfast, one-third after lunch and one-third in the evening after a very small meal. Beyond that, he took a standard high potency vitamin-mineral formula readily available in all drug stores, again far beyond the MDR level.

The theory on which he took these vitamins is that they might revitalize the immune mechanism of his body and increase the vitality in every cell of his body to resist the further development of cancer elsewhere in his body. It is entirely possible that metastases have already spread to other parts of the body, since the type of cancer of the lung that he had had removed spreads through the blood vessels of the body, usually to the lung, the bones, the kidneys and the liver. It was his opinion and his hope that by increasing the vitality of these cells, tissues and organs by proper diet and by the large dosage of vitamins and minerals, his body would be able to contain, control and, perhaps, even destroy such cell spread. There is evidence in the scientific literature he has read that large dosages of vitamin C increase the number of T-lymphocytes in the bloodstream. The T-lymphocytes are a special form of white cell that fight and sometimes destroy cancer cells.

Dr. A. recently brought me up to date on his progress. He had developed a toxic migratory arthralgia from the vitamin A. Niacinamide, which appeared to give relief in the early stages of its trial for control of the symptoms of migratory arthralgia, failed to live up to its promise as time went on, despite increasing the dose from one gram daily to two grams.

It would appear that in his case, even though he had limited his intake of vitamin A to 10,000 I.U. per day when the migratory arthralgia appeared (plus whatever amount there might be in his daily glassful of carrot juice or vitamin A in the form of carotene), the residual symptoms and pathology of migratory arthralgia appeared resistant to the niacinamide.

Symptoms were limited primarily to the ring finger of his right hand and occasionally to the little finger. He did not seek X-ray studies since he knew that metastases would show up primarily in the long bones rather than in the small joints of the hand.

I suggested that he still should be under the care of an oncologist, and follow his instructions. Nevertheless, he preferred to simply follow the revitalization diet and program.

You will learn more about the rest of his diet as we proceed with these consultations. He has always followed precisely the type of diet I have recommended in my previous *Longevity Diet* book and in this present book. Since most such cancer patients are dead within the first six months, the fact that Dr. A. is still alive three and one-half years after surgery without radiation or chemotherapy is hopeful. It does not necessarily prove that his diet, the vitamins and so on have been the deciding factors in this outcome. It is too early to draw any conclusions, but the newer developments with regard to the retinoid do make the result suggestive. He later called to my attention that his previously quite grey hair had turned brown. This was definite evidence, *to him,* of revitalization and even rejuvenation.

At the time of this report, it is three and one-half years since the surgery, and Doctor A. is enjoying the Buddha Walk, and the Buddha Dance, which I will describe in Consultation 6. He most especially finds pleasure and exercise in leading an imaginary orchestra in front of a mirror while listening to music on FM radio. He says this always brings a smile to his face and makes him happy.

The Revitalization Cocktail

Let me recommend to you my "Revitalization Cocktail," which I drink daily. This has been a part of my breakfast for several years.

The Revitalization Cocktail can be prepared in several forms. You can use any mixing device, I use an Osterizer but there are many other commercial blenders that do exactly the same thing. In my personal morning Revitalization Cocktail I place three heaping tablespoonfuls of raw, unprocessed bran, one heaping tablespoonful of raw wheat germ flakes, one heaping tablespoonful of lecithin granules, and one level tablespoonful of brewer's yeast. To this I add three or four grams of vitamin C and four tablets of calcium gluconate with vitamin D. Next, I add one ounce of safflower oil and finish the formula with two-thirds of a glassful of orange juice or apple juice.*

My breakfast consists of the whites of two hardboiled eggs (throwing away the cholesterol-heavy yolks) and the Revitalization Cocktail. On most days, I also have two or three heaping tablespoonfuls of skim milk cottage cheese with a heavy sprinkling of sunflower seeds. This is a very large, very filling, very healthful revitalization breakfast. Another revitalization formula for the cocktail would use skimmed milk as a base in place of the orange juice. This would be the only change.

The cocktail, by itself, is a complete meal since it provides an adequate breakfast quantity of proteins, carbohydrate and polyunsaturated fat. I recommend that if you take this cocktail you could also take 800 I.U. of vitamin E in the d-alpha tocopherol form at the same time. Please note that any vitamin, mineral or other preparation that I suggest, other than food itself, is available

---

*If you need potassium, add one banana to the mixture (or eat it separately).

in all drug stores, and you need not purchase them in health food stores, where the price will be considerably higher. It is not that I have any objection to health food stores; it is merely that I have found no difference between the synthetic vitamins and the so-called "natural" vitamins and minerals.

I must add that at the same time that I take this cocktail and the remainder of my breakfast as described, I also take a high potency vitamin-mineral formula. This formula is also available under several brand names in all pharmacies.

In this way, I start my day with a very filling and yet relatively low-calorie breakfast, and an optimal level of vitamins and minerals.

††*How John R. Reversed Hardening of the Arteries*

John R. was aging prematurely. At forty-three years of age he had evidence of high blood pressure and hardening of the arteries. Even the pulse arteries, at the wrist, revealed hardened areas to the touch.

He was short of breath when walking any distance, lacked energy and suffered from insomnia. He consulted me for bleeding from the rectum; I found internal hemorrhoids and no other pathology. The hemorrhoids responded well to simple injection treatment with a sclerosing agent. However, since the referring physician had told his patient of his cardiovascular condition and had treated him for years without "much good," the physician asked me if I had any suggestions for his patient from the nutritional point of view.

I suggested that he start on the Revitalization Cocktail each morning and be certain that it included one ounce of safflower oil, which is a polyunsaturated oil. I also suggested that he take 800 I.U. (international units) of vitamin E in the d-alpha tocopherol form. Since he was very much overweight (about 60 pounds) I advised him that he eat half-portions at each meal, that his main protein source be fish (preferably ocean fish because of its vanadium content) and that he eliminate all sugars and high-carbohydrate foods such as cakes and candies. I also warned him against his habit of drinking three to five cups of coffee* with each

---

*Coffee, tea, cola, and chocolate have become suspect as possible causes of bowel cancer, and possibly prostate cancer.

meal and suggested that he would do well to stop cigarette smoking. His habit had been one to two packs each day for many years.

His personal physician agreed to have him try this routine, and six months later when he returned for a recheck of his hemorrhoids, I found a totally new man. His blood pressure had returned to normal, his capacity for work and exercise had increased tremendously and he looked about twenty years younger. Also, he no longer had difficulty sleeping.

The High-Protein, Low-Fat, Low-Sugar Diet

Whether you are overweight or underweight, and even if your weight is normal, I strongly suggest that you follow the high-protein, low-fat, low-sugar diet. If you must eat meat, let it be lean meat. If you are a vegetarian, you know that you can obtain all the proteins you need from vegetables. On the other hand, if you are not a vegetarian, I strongly urge you to eat ocean fish rather than meat. Stay away from all processed foods since they contain additives that may have potential dangers. Many processed foods such as breakfast cereals also contain a high level of sugar.

Since 58 percent of the protein you eat and 10 percent of the fats will become sugar in your body in the normal metabolism of those foods, you certainly do not need to add sugar. The simple sugars such as table sugar are particularly dangerous. The complex carbohydrates in vegetables are suitable, but keep the sugar content of your diet down. As for fats, there is evidence that saturated fats may be one cause of hardening of the arteries. Certainly, cholesterol in large amounts like the amount found in egg yolk, should not be part of your diet. Organ meats contain a high level of cholesterol and saturated fats. However, if you enjoy eating liver, a slice of calf's liver once a week should not be detrimental.*

There is scientific proof that you can increase the life-span through diet. I have discussed this at great length in *Longevity Diet*, and have concluded that the life-span can be extended, that

*Experimental studies of nucleosides in liver suggest that they may prevent or control cancer (in mice).

the main factor is diet and that special hope is to be found in avoiding high-calorie foods.

When you limit calories you automatically limit many diseases. When you avoid a high-cholesterol content in your diet and avoid the saturated fats such as those in heavily marbled steak (the most expensive cuts), avoid butter and all other fatty foods, you remove calories and simultaneously reduce the chance of hardening of your arteries.

My best advice is to limit calories, eliminate sugars, starches and saturated fats (as well as cholesterol), and you will be on your way toward a revitalized body and a happier life.

††How Eleanor W. Reduced Weight and Increased Vitality—The Easy Way

This patient, at 34 years of age, was not only very much overweight (approximately 47 pounds for her height and age), but also found that she tired easily and had lost interest in life generally. Her obvious loss of vitality could have been connected with her equally obvious increase in weight. However, there were also emotional problems to be considered. Her first husband had died three years before, and the experience had left her very depressed. Her only interest was in playing cards with her few women friends. Since they were married, they were attempting to find another husband for her—unsuccessfully. It was obvious that in her depressed state, overeating was the remedy she had chosen to satisfy her loss of interest in life.

I told her that the best solution was to lose weight as quickly as possible and to begin seeing other men as soon as she felt that she had regained her figure and her desire for living. The natural consequence would be increased vitality and, ultimately, greater satisfaction with life. This, I said to her, was the easy way. The hard way would be to see a psychiatrist over a period of months or years, after which she would possibly lose her depression and regain her desire to live.

She chose to follow my instructions. I placed her on the high-protein, low-fat, low-sugar diet and advised her to take a high potency vitamin-mineral formula daily.

I told her to take the Revitalization Cocktail, as described, each morning. That was to be her entire breakfast. Lunch was to be three tablespoonfuls of cottage cheese with a heavy sprinkling of sunflower seeds. This was to be followed, in turn, by another five grams of vitamin C in a glass of orange juice. Her evening meal was to consist of a very large salad of mixed greens, followed by broiled or steamed fish (preferably ocean fish) and cooked vegetables. She was not to drink coffee or tea.

She followed my advice precisely, rapidly lost her excess weight and regained her former attractive figure. This inspired her to buy a new wardrobe, and soon she was happily meeting men who interested her and in whom she became interested. She had reduced weight and increased her vitality the easy way.

Food for the Mind

Please remember that in my concept, your "mind" is not only in your brain and the rest of your nervous system, but also in each cell, each tissue, each organ of your body. Obviously then, food for your body is also food for your mind. But equally as obvious, your central nervous system has special requirements from a nutritional point of view. And each "mind" is unique in its requirements. Beyond that, since we are what we eat and what we think, "food," when we are speaking of the mind, involves both our thought patterns and our eating patterns. It is my personal belief that the Revitalization Cocktail and the other suggestions that I have made and will continue to make throughout these consultations will provide your body-mind complex with the best possible food for your body and for your mind.

There are many physicians who are coming to believe that depression and other emotional disturbances, including schizophrenia and allied conditions, are to some degree benefited by appropriate nutrition. My practice did not include the treatment of such disorders, but it is obvious that every person has times of depression and times during which the stress is so great that they appear on the point of a mental-emotional breakdown. Therefore, I have had to consider for such patients the appropriate nutrition intakes that would be antistress and hopefully antidepressive. The next case history illustrates this type of approach to a patient who was suffering stress-depression.

††*How Ruth C. Conquered Physical Depression—A Simple Formula for Rapid Relief*

Ruth C. was forty-three years of age, suffered from the stress of an unhappy marriage and had an overactive large bowel. Her emotional disturbance and stress had caused the reaction of the large bowel in terms of overactivity and recurrent bouts of what had been termed by her family physician as "colitis." A thorough examination by X-ray study of the large bowel and a sigmoidoscopy revealed that there were no ulcerations and there was no evidence of inflammatory disease of the large bowel. What we were seeing was a stress reaction.

I placed Ruth on an appropriate diet to improve digestion and bowel action (see Consultation 3), and advised her that I believed she might be helped—even in terms of her depression—once the bowel was under control through the intake of appropriate amounts of certain vitamins. The vitamins I particularly recommended were thiamine (B1) and ascorbic acid (vitamin C). I suggested that she take at least 100 mg. of thiamine, and at least two grams each day of ascorbic acid. However, I cautioned Ruth that she might have a reaction to the ascorbic acid that would be distressing and that the dosage should be reduced if she did have diarrhea and/or flatulence. Thiamine, I told her, might produce nausea in large dosage. I suggested a stress-level vitamin-mineral combination to start with, since this would include both of these vitamins in relatively small dosage compared with the ultimate level that I thought she might need.

Ruth C's physical-emotional (body-mind) depression was rapidly relieved, beginning with the alleviation of the overactive bowel and continuing with what appeared to be an actual rejuvenation. New vitality was evident in her appearance, in her bearing and in her relaxed control. Her intake of specific vitamins had indeed proved to be a simple formula for rapid relief of a physical depression.

††*And now, In Summary . . .*

1. **During our first consultation, you have learned a little about me and a great deal about my concepts as they relate to the mind-body.**
2. **You have learned that my purpose is to treat the mind-body as a single unit, not simply to treat a disease.**

3. You know now that there are multiple causes for each disease, and that you—as a human being—require treatment of the total mind-body.

4. I have advised you—since you are totally unique—to consult your physician before entering upon any form of self-treatment. You are not a doctor, and this book may not have the precise answer you need. My objective is to show you how to slow aging and restore vitality to aging cells, tissues and organs. However, your physician will need to make the first evaluation of your general health and of your body functions.

5. You have learned how cigarette smoke can cause cancer of the lung, even if you are a nonsmoker. Be cautious when you sit in a theatre or an airplane, always choosing the non-smoking section. If you are now a smoker, make the choice between life and death. The choice is yours.

6. I have told you of research now going on related to nutrition in the prevention of cancer and nutrition in the prolongation of life in patients with terminal cancer. The final answer to this terrible problem has not yet been found. If you suspect cancer, or if the diagnosis has been made, do not attempt to treat yourself. Try to obtain the advice and treatment of a cancer specialist—an oncologist.

7. You have learned how to prepare the Revitalization Cocktail in two different forms. You have also learned my personal breakfast Revitalization Cocktail and the other foods that I eat in the morning.

8. You have learned how proper diet can reverse hardening of the arteries (atherosclerosis) and improve cardiac function.

9. You know about the high-protein, low-fat, low-sugar diet and what it will do for your heart, arteries and life-span and how it can effect a revitalization of distressed cells, tissues and organs.

10. You have also learned that it is sometimes possible to help those who have physical depression by restoring vitality to the body-mind. We will have much more to say about this in later consultations as it relates to self-destructive, stressful thought patterns already in most minds and how to get rid of them.

11. Finally, I have talked to you about food for the mind both in terms of nutrition and in terms of mind content.

With your doctor's approval you may now start on the road toward a revitalized energy bank. I would suggest that you learn to think happy thoughts. Stop the "gloom-and-doom" thoughts. Positive thinking should be in terms of revitalization, better health and longer life. Keep telling yourself, "healthier and healthier, happier and happier, better and better." Do your best to live life one moment at a time and keep life simple. You can only live *now*.

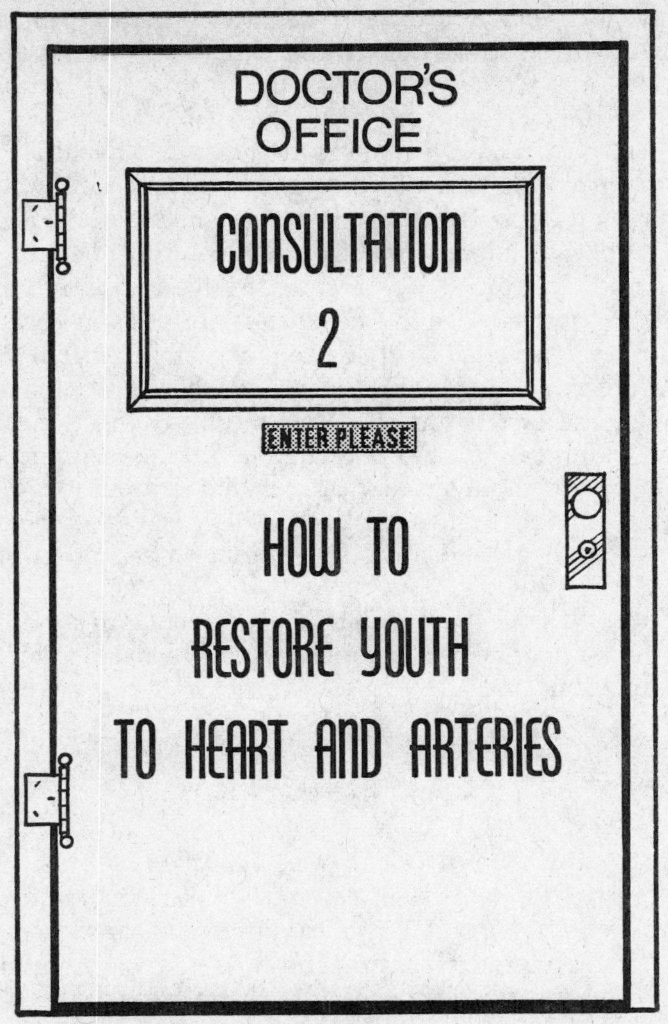

DOCTOR'S
OFFICE
CONSULTATION
2
ENTER PLEASE
HOW TO
RESTORE YOUTH
TO HEART AND ARTERIES

When your heart functions normally and when your arteries are not blocked by hardened plaques of cholestrol, your blood supply can flow normally to the cells, tissues and organs of your body. When your blood supply is reduced by such blockage, spasms of the arteries or irregularities of heartbeat, then your tissues do not receive proper nutrition and your cells, tissues and organs no longer function normally. Premature aging sets in and stroke or heart attack may result. During this consultation I would like to tell you about the "magic" minerals, the gift of the sea, polyunsaturated versus saturated fats and the general importance of diet in overcoming or preventing disease of your heart and arteries. I believe we can safely say that you are as old as your arteries, as old as your heart.

You will have taken a major step toward a healthier future and toward revitalization of your entire body when you have learned how to control the dangerous deposits in your arteries. To function properly the heart muscle must receive adequate blood from its coronary arteries, which actually feed the heart muscle with its blood supply. When one of these arteries is obstructed, the heart muscle supplied by that artery actually dies. The clotting and closing of the artery is known as a coronary thrombosis, and the death of the heart muscle is technically called "myocardial infarction." You need not be concerned about the technical terms. All you need to know is that by proper diet, proper exercise and proper food for the mind and body, this disease of heart and arteries can be postponed for many years and can often even be prevented.

It is not too late. I am not talking about taking medicines, although you should certainly consult your physician in any case. I am talking about diet alone or diet combined with proper exercise.

The Magic Minerals

Extensive and careful research by William H. Strain, Ph.D., of the University of Rochester's School of Medicine showed that vanadium, a mineral found in the drinking water of some areas of the Southwest United States, prevented heart and cardiovascular problems in the people who used it in those areas. These are the areas that were once covered by the ancient Permian Seas (about 200 million years ago), and vanadium appears to be the factor in those waters that prevents and controls heart disease. The "magic" mineral, vanadium, seems to check and prevent cholesterol development in the body. The less cholesterol there is in the bloodstream, the less accumulation there will be of cholesterol in our artery walls. Dr. Strain goes even further and tells us that "proper dietary intake of vanadium may give lower cholesterol content to the skin, reduces the incidence of gall stones and lessens accumulation of cholesterol in the arterial walls."

Zinc is another mystery mineral that seems to be essential for both the repair and growth of our body tissues. There is also some possibility that it may be important to gall bladder function as well as to the structure of our arteries.

Dr. Strain found widespread deficiencies of both zinc and vanadium in the average American diet. There is proof that the Permian Seas that once covered much of the South Central and Mountain States contained large amounts of both zinc and vanadium. People who live in those areas have a lower death rate than average from heart and blood vessel disease. It is important that you benefit from this knowledge by including both zinc and vanadium in your diet.

The Gift of the Sea

The gift of the sea includes much more than vanadium and zinc. However, for our present consultation, let us concentrate on these two elements. If you learn to enjoy sardines and herrings you will obtain an adequate amount of both vanadium and zinc. Indeed, all ocean fish contain vanadium, the content varying with the species. Some contain both vanadium and zinc, especially sardines and herrings. Eat fish regularly—the Scandinavians do, and this may be a factor in their healthy bodies, great vitality and possibly in their longevity. Remember that when you lower cholesterol levels, your arteries will become younger and your heart will function better. If you take only 3 1/2 ounces of sardines you will provide your body with 560 milligrams of potassium as well as vanadium and zinc.

The most important researcher on stress is Dr. Hans Selye of the University of Montreal. He has found that under certain experimental conditions the heart muscle dies as a result of deficiencies in magnesium and potassium. Both of these minerals are obviously essential for proper heart muscle function. Dr. Selye's conclusion from these experiments is that prevention or treatment can be effective when magnesium and potassium are taken daily, and that they may be the ultimate answer for all types of heart muscle death.

There have been confirmations from other researchers, and we could fill these pages simply by listing the extensive number of papers that have been written in support of this concept. The "magic" minerals are magic indeed, they may save your life, revitalize your heart and arteries and add years to your lifespan.

You Must Have the "Magic" Minerals Every Day

We cannot store minerals in our body to a sufficient degree to prevent heart and artery disease. Therefore, we must eat appropriate foods each day in order to obtain these necessary minerals. I strongly urge that you drink bottled hard water and avoid the water that comes from your faucet unless you live in the South Central and Mountain States where the waters naturally contain large amounts of both vanadium and zinc. I urge that you drink at least six to eight glasses of water a day to avoid the drying out of body tissues. Remember, your body is largely water. It is interesting to note that about 30 percent of the fluid in our bodies has essentially the same composition as dilute seawater.

It not only important to obtain a sufficient quantity of the appropriate "magic" minerals in your diet, but they must be in proper balance. This is especially important when we consider calcium and magnesium, which must be kept at balanced levels. When you take the Revitalization Cocktail each morning, you will be obtaining a balanced level of certain minerals and vitamins. When you add a high potency vitamin-mineral formula (easily obtainable in any pharmacy) to this, you will be providing yourself with adequate safeguards against a deficiency of both minerals and vitamins. You will be going still further in terms of the revitalization effect of the cocktail combined with the vitamin-mineral formula. In our fourth consultation I will be telling you more about the soybean protein and the Revitalization Cocktail. I will also tell you about the magic of selenium, another trace mineral of enormous importance.

Polyunsaturated Versus Saturated Fats

Physicians seem to be about equally divided on the question of the importance of polyunsaturated versus saturated fats in the prevention of heart and artery disease. We do know, for an absolute fact, that unsaturated fats are essential in our diet. When you take the Revitalization Cocktail you will have taken soybean lecithin, which is an important polyunsaturated fat. Lecithin is an emulsifying agent that tends to actually dissolve deposits of cholesterol. Most of the early research on lecithin was done by Dr. L. M. Morrison, who subsequently reported that cholesterol levels in the blood of twelve patients were lowered effectively when they took about one ounce of lecithin each day for three months.

Start eating half-portions. There is an old saying: Half the food you eat keeps you alive while the other half kills you. So leave the half that kills you on your plate. Polyunsaturated fats will reduce your desire for food. Thus, the polyunsaturated fats in lecithin and in safflower oil will help you reach your goal of half-portion eating. This is an important function of the polyunsaturated fats. Combined with your desire to restore youth and to revitalize your body (a desire that will keep you on the right path as described in this series of consultations), the polyunsaturated fats in your Revitalization Cocktail will actually turn off the "appestat" mechanism at the base of your brain that signals hunger. The combination is very effective.

Indeed, if you are anything like my patients and myself, the Revitalization Cocktail alone will be a very satisfying breakfast. When you add the sunflower seeds (also high in polyunsaturated fats) and skimmed milk cottage cheese, as well as the whites of two hard-boiled eggs, you have a well-balanced, excellent, healthful, revitalizing meal. Believe me, you will not be anxious for more food until five or six hours have passed.

The Cholesterol Puzzle

Please remember that cholesterol is an essential element in the body. We cannot live without it. It makes up an important part of our most vital organs and tissues. Recent reports have revealed that cholesterol is carried by more than six different chemicals, and some of these protect against heart disease. This seems confusing, and I ask you to bear with me for a few moments. Perhaps we can, to some degree, resolve the controversy related to saturated and polyunsaturated fats, cholesterol, and so on, concerning heart disease and hardening of the arteries.

The new studies do confirm the great importance of avoiding a heavy-fat diet. When we combine a diet that contains too much fat (most especially the saturated fats) with a lack of exercise, we have the basic elements for heart disease. A recent report during an American Heart Association meeting showed that there are "various cholesterol-carrying substances that play an important role in determining whether or not the fat in your diet will cause heart and artery disease." There are three types of lipoproteins that carry the cholesterol around in our blood stream. One type is called VLDL—very low density lipoprotein. This type of lipoprotein transports triglycerides. Now where do triglycerides come from? When you eat a large amount of carbohydrates (sugars) and you eat too much (excessive calories), these triglycerides form.

The next step occurs when these triglycerides leave the carrier VLDLs at various fatty deposits in your body. Here, they are converted to another type of lipoprotein, LDL (low density lipoprotein). These low density lipoproteins (LDLs) are composed of cholesterol in their core, and they then carry cholesterol from your liver to your various cells and tissues. It would seem, then, that the cholesterol in your liver is the result of both your diet and synthesis by the liver. I understand that this may sound very complicated to you, but you will not need to remember anything except the conclusions. However, it will be of interest to some of you and to physician readers in the better understanding of the cholesterol / heart attack / atherosclerosis puzzle.

There is a third kind of lipoprotein, HDL which is a high density lipoprotein. It functions to remove excess cholesterol from your tissues and return it to your liver. The liver than excretes it. The importance of all this is that the HDLs (high density lipoproteins) are considered in theory to be the major factor in removing cholesterol from your artery walls. Since deposit of cholesterol on the walls of your arteries is the main factor in hardening of your arteries (atherosclerosis), anything that clears these deposits will restore flexibility to your arteries and youth to your tissues. No doubt, clearing these deposits will also prolong life. Thus, it would appear that these high density lipoproteins (HDLs) are the important factors in protecting us from heart and artery disease.

Framingham, Massachusetts is a town in which practically the entire population has been studied for heart and artery problems for a very long time. A report by Dr. William P. Castelzi, Director of Laboratories for the Framingham study, advised the American Heart Association that those townspeople who were found to have high levels of HDL-cholesterol in their blood have been less subject to heart disease than those who have high levels of LDL. It would appear, then, that the lipoprotein-cholesterol puzzle has many parts. It is not simply the amount of cholesterol that you consume, or perhaps even the amount of saturated fats, but the levels of the various carrier lipoproteins in your body that determine whether or not a high level of cholesterol will indeed cause a heart attack.

The Framingham research showed that women before menopause have higher levels of the protective HDL-cholesterol than men of the same age. This may account for the lower national rate of heart disease in women than in men below the age of fifty. It is also interesting to note that regular exercise, especially strenuous exercise, increases the HDL levels in male bloodstreams.

It is also important for us to realize, however, that if you are overweight you will most likely have a lower level of the HDL carrier. When you lose weight, as you will when you are following the Revitalization Cocktail and half-portion diet, the protective HDL level will usually increase. This appears to be the mechanism for the reduction of cholesterol in heart and arteries as well as in the blood stream, when weight reduction occurs.

Still more recent studies on cholesterol show that there is a fourth-type of lipoprotein, also of high density, called HDL-c to distinguish it from the previously discovered HDL. The newly discovered form of HDL-c acts like the low density lipoprotein (LDL), and is attracted to receptors on the surface of our body cells, delivering cholesterol into these cells. This is precisely what the low density lipoproteins do, but the HDL-c seems to do it more actively than the LDL. Obviously, when cholesterol enters a cell it can cause hardening of the lining of the walls of the arteries.

Now we come to the practical application of this knowledge. The cholesterol in egg yolks is a source of potential danger to your arteries. In each egg there is at least 250 milligrams of cholesterol. I advise eating only the whites of hard-boiled eggs and throwing away the egg-yolk. The American Heart Association, and many physicians, advise that we take no more than 300 milligrams of cholesterol each day, from all sources, including both dairy and meat products. Since we now know that both low density lipoproteins (LDL) and even high density lipoproteins of the HDL-c variety act to introduce cholesterol into the cells, causing atherosclerosis, the new research further stresses the great importance of limiting the amount of cholesterol in your diet.

Once again, if you limit your cholesterol intake by removing the fatty meats from your diet and eating only the whites of hard-boiled eggs, your chance of developing hardening of the arteries is greatly decreased.

Naturally, there will be a variation in each person depending upon the types of lipoproteins in each individual's bloodstream. There are some people who, through genetic factors, have an unusually high HDL level and a high total cholesterol count and still live long lives free of heart disease, well into their eighties and nineties. Now what does all this mean to you? It means that when your physician sends you for a blood cholesterol study, he should also have a study made of the level of your lipoproteins. Obviously, if you have a high HDL level, that may be the reason for your high cholesterol level. In that case, you may not need any form of treatment or alteration of diet. But don't count on it. This does not appear to be very common. Avoid the diet with large amounts of sugars and saturated fats. Avoid the steak houses and hamburger stands. There is even some evidence that a high-fat diet may be responsible for certain cancers of the large bowel, to make things even worse.

If you eat large amounts of saturated fats, as most people do in the United States, your liver will make more VLDLs and LDLs, and you will be well on your way toward hardening of the arteries and a heart attack. Your liver will make less of the protective HDLs. On the positive side of the longevity ledger, we should make a note that the polyunsaturated fats promote cholesterol transport by the HDLs rather than by the LDLs and VLDLs.

The Final Conclusion on the Fat Controversy

I urge you to avoid cholesterol in your diet. I urge you to avoid saturated fats, and to protect yourself with a relatively small amount of the polyunsaturated fats such as those in the Revitalization Cocktail. You need not remember any of the details above, but if you consult a physician, I urge you to request that he not only arrange for a blood cholesterol level report but a study of the blood lipoproteins. He can even do this himself by putting a sample of your blood in the refrigerator and looking at it the next day. If the sample shows a cloudiness throughout, this will mean a large amount of HDL. If the top layer is creamy, that is due to the LDLs. If there is a very small band over the LDL, that band is

VLDL. But the laboratory that does the study of your total blood picture can make a very precise and detailed analysis for your physician and for you.

One final note of caution. There are animal studies that show the importance of having sufficient oxygen in the blood since a lower level of oxygen than normal increases the amount of LDL-cholesterol in the experimental tissue cells. This means that you had better stop smoking cigarettes if you really wish to reduce your chances of hardening of the arteries and a heart attack.

A recent study in Finland showed that the very high heart attack rate in that country (the highest in the world) could be reduced by 40 percent by eliminating high blood cholesterol, high blood pressure and smoking. The Finns concluded that these were the main causes of heart disease, so they passed laws forbidding smoking on public transportation, in public buildings, and even in many private offices. They urged a switch to skimmed milk, change from butter to margarine, made sausages with a 25 percent mushroom content in place of the heavy fat and started a major campaign to persuade housewives to bring fresh vegetables into the diet of the home.

Exercise for Revitalization

I will have much to say in our sixth consultation about the importance of exercise and various methods of exercise for those who want to turn back the clock. I will also describe isometric pre-sleep exercise in our seventh consultation. There is no question that those who practice a regular pattern of hard physical exercise or work will lower their risk of dying from heart and artery disease. A twenty-two year study of 3,600 longshoremen in San Francisco proves this. To turn back the clock and to revitalize your body, I therefore suggest that you begin a graduated program of exercise. Begin with the mildest form of exercise, simply walking. Do not overdo it. When you are short of breath, stop. Let your walking, at first, be at a slow pace. Gradually increase the pace, but never to the point where you are short of breath. Increase the pace and the time only in terms of an absence of stress on the heart and lungs. Let shortness of breath be your guide. When you feel tired or short of breath, stop. Stop instantly. Resume your walk at a slower pace.

While you are walking, repeat to yourself the following formula for revitalization, "Younger and younger, younger and younger, younger and younger." Say this with each step, and you will soon find that your steps take on an added vitality and bounce. You will be programming both your body and your mind—food for the mind and food for the body—toward slower aging and restoration of youth.

The combination of the contents of the Revitalization Cocktail, the half-portion diet, the elimination of fats in your diet, the avoidance of tobacco, the elimination of coffee, the supplementary vitamin-mineral capsule formula and—as a final point—appropriate exercise, with a programmed message of "Younger and younger, younger and younger, younger and younger" will increase your chances for slower aging, restoration of youth and prolongation of life.

††*How Wallace L. Overcame Angina*

Wallace L. had been suffering from pain in the chest after the slightest exertion for the last three of his 63 years. He had consulted eminent cardiologists and had been advised properly, without a doubt. He had been given the important drugs available during those times for the control of pain. However, he had obviously never followed instructions with regard to nutrition; perhaps he had never been given any.

He was overweight by 48 pounds for his age and height. He had been told to reduce but, apparently, had either never followed the instructions or had never received instructions that suited his temperament. I told him that unless he lost these excess pounds of fat, the chances of controlling his angina without drugs—or even with them—was not very good. Indeed, his lifespan would be very much shortened if he did not lose the excess weight.

I told him about the half-portion diet and the enormous importance of avoiding sugars, fats of all types (with the exception of the polyunsaturated fat that he would have in his Revitalization Cocktail), salt (since this tends to damage the kidneys and raise the blood pressure), cigarettes and coffee.

He lived an active life as a stock broker, and I advised him that it was important for him to practice walking in a very graduated fashion. The pattern of walking is the one that I have just described. He was to repeat to himself as he walked.

"Healthier and healthier, healthier and healthier, every day in every way, healthier and healthier." This served two purposes. First, it emptied the mind of distressing thoughts and replaced the stress-causing anxieties of his past with a health-building form of programming of the mind that has its effects on every cell, every tissue and every organ.

I explained to him that since the anxieties of the troubled past, the fears of the future and his present anxieties would ordinarily be in the forefront of his mind, we would have to quiet his mind and replace such stressful thoughts with a health-building formula. He understood clearly and followed my instructions to a T. The slow walking, combined with the stress-erasing formula and the positive health-building content of that formula, relaxes the muscles of the body (including the muscles of the arteries of the body) and provides a healthful background for the revitalization of all cells, all tissues and all organs.

Whereas, before beginning the program I have just outlined, Wallace could walk no more than half a block without needing to stop until the dreadful pain and pressure in his left chest diminished or disappeared, he gradually came to the point where he would walk several blocks and then several miles without experiencing angina.

During this time, the weight loss, the Revitalization Cocktail, the vitamin-mineral formula that I have described (together with 800 I.U. vitamin E) and the new outlook on life that developed all combined to totally revitalize, reenergize and almost rejuvenate this man.

Particularly Important Vitamins for Long Life

I consider it important that each one of us have an adequate supply of all vitamins. That is why I use a large dosage of vitamin C in the Revitalization Cocktail and advise that the patients supplement their diet with a high-potency vitamin-mineral formula. However, I would like to say a word about the controversial vitamin E. It is my considered opinion that an inadequate amount of vitamin E in the diet may be fundamental in the development of heart disease and atherosclerosis. I therefore urge that everybody, as a simple preventive measure, take 800 I.U. (international units) of vitamin E in the d-alpha tocopherol form each day. Vitamin E and vitamin C are antioxidants. There is a theory that it is best not to oxidize the polyunsaturated fats since this peroxidation causes what is called "free radical production." Radiation also causes free radical formation and these free radicals are considered by some expert researchers in longevity to be a cause of aging.

Therefore, when taking the polyunsaturates, I recommend both vitamin E in relatively substantial amounts and vitamin C in large dosage. The vitamin C is in the Revitalization Cocktail. The vitamin E is taken in capsule form. It would appear, on the basis of some reports, that those people suffering from hypertension should not take large amounts of vitamin E; 800 I.U. is a safe upper limit. Incidentally, selenium is also an antioxidant.

It seems to me, that from a practical point of view, the combination of vitamin E and ascorbic acid would be effective in preventing premature aging and in reversing the aging process, by the prevention of peroxidation, as well as by their other reported beneficial effects on cells, tissues and organs of the body.

The most important vitamins and minerals appear to be vitamin A (at least 10,000 units as a daily supplement), vitamin D (500 units), ascorbic acid, (10 grams in three divided doses of equal amounts, one dose after each meal), thiamine (at least 2 mg., and the same amount for riboflavin), pyridoxine (3-5 mg.), pantothenate (20 mg.), niacinamide (20 mg.), vitamin B^{12} (5 mcg.), choline (100 mg.) and inositol (100 mg). As for the minerals, I would suggest calcium in the amount of at least 300 mg. (always with vitamin D), magnesium (100 mg.), zinc (5 mg.), iron (10 mg.), cobalt (.1 mg.), copper (1 mg.), iodine (.1 mg.), molybdenum (12 mg.) and manganese (1 mg.).

If you take any of the high-potency vitamin-mineral formulas presently available on the market, you will receive an appropriate dosage of most of these vitamins and minerals, but you will have to take a supplementary additional quanity of both vitamin C and vitamin E if you are following my revitalization formula.

Please remember that I am not advising toxic levels of any vitamins, and if you are concerned—as you should be—about appropriate levels of vitamin A and vitamin D in terms of appropriate dosage, you should consult your physician.

My objective in writing this book, in holding these consultations and in relating the case histories is to illustrate to you the importance of nutrition in the health and vitality of your entire body.

The food you eat and the thoughts you think will determine how long you will live, the degree of vitality you will enjoy during your lifetime, the rapidity of the aging process and how happy your life will be. None of this can be guaranteed. All of it depends upon how well you understand the mind-body approach to aging and restoration of youth and how well you apply the total formula as it relates to both mind and body as a single unit.

††*How John B. Controlled and Reversed Intermittent Claudication*

When I first saw John B., he had been to several physicians for the treatment of intermittent claudication. This is a condition in which there is spasm of the blood vessels of the legs, resulting in hardening of the muscles of the legs and pain resulting from a lack of blood supply to those muscles. When walking, John was often forced to stop where he was and wait until the spasm within the walls of the blood vessels released and the circulation improved. He could then walk on for a further distance before it occurred again. In many ways, this is comparable to the angina pectoris that causes severe spasm of the arteries of the heart and pain in the chest.

It has been claimed by Dr. Shute of Canada that vitamin E., in large dosage, would control and reverse this condition. Work at one of the major clinics in the United States seems to confirm this and so reported in the scientific medical literature. Since physicians had treated John B. with various medications which proved ineffective, I suggested the same type of vitamin E program for him. I asked him to gradually increase walking, associating this with the brain-clearing and health-producing repeated thought, "Better and better, healthier and healthier, younger and younger." I recommended 800 I.U. of vitamin E at the outset, and later I increased this to 1,600 and then 2,000 I.U. since the patient was not having any increase in blood pressure. (With elevated blood pressure, it is probably best to keep vitamin E dosage at or below the 800 I.U. level.)

The combination of the Revitalization Cocktail, the revitalization diet and the relatively large dosage of special vitamins gradually produced a reversal of John B's claudication and finally—over a period of six months—gave him complete freedom from spasms as long as he did not attempt running. Running produced a spasm, but the spasm quickly reversed itself when he paused and relaxed.

Even more remarkable was the change in John's general appearance and the obvious revitalization of his entire body and mind. He looked much more youthful, his walk now had the springy bounce of youth and his face radiated confidence in place of his previous stress.

††*What Onions Did for Dr. Jones*

Dr. Jones had referred many patients to me over the course of approximately thirty years and knew of my special interest in nutrition. He was overweight, although he advised all his patients to keep their weight "down." It was a case of "Do as I say and not as I do." Dr. Jones was a surgeon and was apparently always under stress, not only at the hospital but at home. He had been considering divorce for a long time.

He consulted me on the matter of nutrition as it related to what he called "stress headaches." These were very much like typical migraine headaches; severe, on one side of the head and sometimes incapacitating. I told him of the experiments on biofeedback in which the patient learned how to warm his hands or feet by controlling the flow of his blood to those extremities and about how this relieved migraine. These experiments had been done at various clinics, especially at the Menninger Foundation in Topeka, Kansas, a psychiatric clinic. Biofeedback training uses an instrument to record and to show a patient's stress either in terms of the measurement of his brain waves or in terms of the measurement of perspiration on his fingertips. I told Dr. Jones that he might not need the instruments to use biofeedback technique. He might obtain biofeedback benefits by simply plunging his hands or his feet into a container of hot water while relaxing. I suggested that he do this while sitting back in a chair, closing his eyes, letting all his muscles go limp and loose and simply saying to himself, "Better and better, healthier and healthier, happier and happier."

It was important, I advised him, to relax both body and mind, since they are one entity. In his case—the family stress being what it was—it would be best if he had a private room where he could relax without interference. Naturally, I also placed him on the Revitalization Cocktail and the longevity diet, told him that he must give up his habit of constantly smoking cigarettes and advised him that he would also be wise to forego his usual three cups of coffee with each meal. Finally, I informed him that onions contain selenium and that if he didn't mind eating whole onions, it would be helpful to him to increase the level of selenium in his blood stream, since this is an important antioxidant, comparable to vitamin E and vitamin C. He said that he loved onions and would follow my instructions.

Jokingly, I said to him "Eating onions will also reduce stress for you." "How do you account for that?" he responded. My answer was, "They will keep people away from you." He laughed, but realized the importance of this in terms of his awkward—to say the least—family life. I told him that he could also obtain selenium in combination with vitamin E in a health food store. I knew of no pharmacies that produced this particular combination, but it was available in health food stores.

Dr. Jones followed my instructions closely, and within a relatively short time, he began to show a greatly improved capacity for work and a capacity to handle the stress of his home life as well as his work. Within six months, his entire personality appeared to have changed, and I told him that I believed the onions were indeed working, "by keeping him away from people." He laughed, and shook his head affirmatively. Within six to eight months Dr. Jones no longer suffered migraine headaches, and seemed to be much happier in his work and with his family. I never did ask him whether his wife learned to love onions as much as he did.

††*How Stuart L. Lowered Blood Pressure and Prevented a Stroke*

Stuart L. was in his mid-sixties, with a blood pressure level very close to that which results in a rupture of the blood vessel in the brain, commonly called a "stroke." His physician had prescribed the usual medications to lower blood pressure and to take as a diuretic. But he had not advised Stuart L. on how to reduce stress and how to overcome his obesity.

Stuart L. was referred to me for the treatment of bleeding hemorrhoids, but I advised him that it was not desirable to operate until his blood pressure was reduced. I told him that when his blood pressure was reduced it was entirely possible that the hemorrhoids would cease bleeding. I also told him that the bleeding could be serving as a life-saving mechanism at the present time, as nose bleeds do for other patients with high blood pressure. It is much better to bleed from the bowel through dilated hemorrhoids or from the nose through dilated blood vessels in the nose than to have the elevated pressure rupture a blood vessel in the brain.

I placed Stuart L. on the Revitalization Cocktail and provided him with the instructions for an appropriate low-fat, low-sugar, high-protein diet without coffee or tea. He was a non-smoker, fortunately, so we did not have that problem. Stuart L. needed to relax, and I showed him relaxation methods comparable to those described above, and those you will find described in your sixth and seventh consultations.

He was told to practice relaxation three times a day, while lying down. He was to relax awhile in the morning immediately upon awakening, whenever it was convenient for him to lie down in the afternoon and before going to sleep. I taught him how to talk to his muscles, from head to toe, simply saying "relax toes," "relax feet" and so on, until his entire body was so instructed and relaxed. Stuart usually found that this relaxation became very deep and helped him to sleep quickly and easily in the evening. In the afternoon, since he was fortunate enough to have the time, his relaxation led to a one- or two-hour nap. The meditation formula that I advised him to say to himself was, "Healthier and healthier, every day in every way." He was to repeat this as soon as he was completely relaxed and until he fell asleep or returned to his normal activity.

Stuart took slow walks, on my advice, with repetition of the same formula, for at least twenty or thirty minutes each day, regardless of the weather, unless it was heavy rain or snow. Under those weather conditions, he practiced the same exercise by walking back and forth through his living room for the same length of time. The result was remarkably good, his blood pressure came down to very close to normal, and the bleeding from his hemorrhoids stopped completely. I had the great pleasure and satisfaction of a telephone call from Stuart L's physician, asking me how I had accomplished this "miracle." Naturally, I told him precisely what I had done, and he gratefully said, "I do appreciate it, and will now use your techniques for most of my patients."

††How to Do It Yourself Now!

1. If you have not already done so, start on the Revitalization Cocktail and my breakfast program (see the first consultation).
2. Start immediately on the high-protein, low-fat, low-sugar diet.
3. If you are a smoker, stop immediately. If you drink coffee, stop right now. You will save money, your health and perhaps your life.
4. Avoid meat, especially the so-called "better cuts" of steak, since they have a very high saturated-fat content. Avoid butter.
5. Eat ocean fish every day, if possible.
6. Take a high-potency vitamin-mineral capsule each day, preferably with your breakfast Revitalization Cocktail. Take 800 I.U. vitamin E daily.
7. If you like onions as much as I do, follow Dr. Jones's example, and eat whole onions. A simple lunch might consist of a tin of tuna and a whole onion.
8. Learn to relax in the way I have just described, and—wherever possible—practice relaxation in the morning, afternoon and before sleeping.
9. Use the stress-reducing formulas that I have described in this consultation such as "Better and better, healthier and healthier, happier and happier" at every possible opportunity during the course of the day.
10. Use this formula while taking a twenty or thirty minute walk. It will empty your mind, relax your body and improve your health as the combination provides "food" for your mind and body.

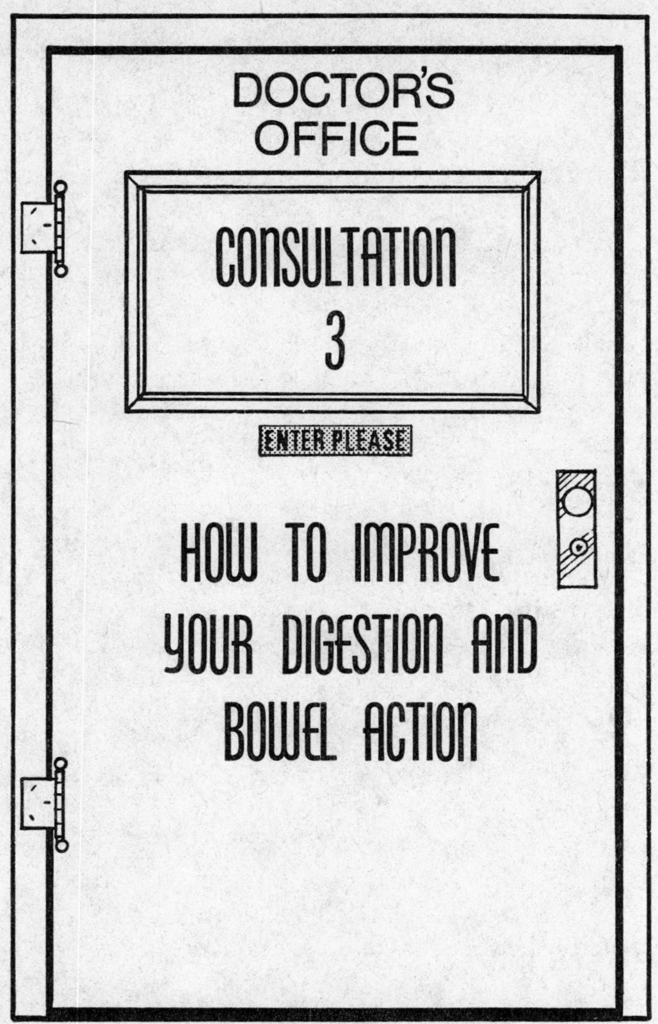

DOCTOR'S
OFFICE
CONSULTATION
3
ENTER PLEASE
HOW TO IMPROVE
YOUR DIGESTION AND
BOWEL ACTION

The Magic Secret of Bran

During forty years of practice of medicine, most of which has been directed toward the gastrointestinal tract, I have never prescribed laxatives or cathartics for any patient. Whenever there was a choice between drugs and diet, if diet would do as much or more for the patient than drugs, I preferred to advise proper nutrition.

Constipation is a very common problem. In the vast majority of cases, the cause is improper nutrition. As I have said to some patients, "If you don't put the proper food in one end of the intestinal tract, you will not have a proper bowel movement coming out of the other end of the intestinal tract." In my long experience in treating constipation and other problems of the bowel, I have found that bran has been the most effective treatment. You will recall that the Revitalization Cocktail contains two heaping tablespoons of bran—this will be most effective for the average person. If this is insufficient to relieve your constipation, I would suggest that you take a third tablespoon of bran with or after lunch. That will usually be enough. Occasionally, however, a particularly obstinate problem may require still another tablespoon of bran with or after your evening meal.

What we are dealing with in constipation is a *fiber deficiency* in the diet, and bran is a *high-fiber* natural food. When you put it in your mixing device with the other ingredients of the Revitalization Cocktail, you will be converting rough bran into fine bran. If you prefer, however, you can take it separately, simply by sprinkling it over your skimmed milk cottage cheese at breakfast time. Do not *think* of bran as "roughage" in the sense that it is "rough." Since bran absorbs water, it becomes anything but rough as soon as it enters the stomach. Some people require much less bran, and you may start with a single heaping tablespoonful of bran in your cocktail, especially if you find that the bran causes excessive passage of gas from the bowel.

There are other "high residue" foods you should also eat. What we are after is a high-residue, high-roughage diet, and you should regularly eat fresh vegetables or lightly cooked vegetables, fresh fruits and high-fiber grains. You will not find much high-fiber grain in ordinary breakfast cereal, though. Instead, you will get a high content of sugar in such cereals, which is *not* included in our revitalization program.

One of the earliest writers on the importance of bran was a surgeon, Captain Cleave of the British Royal Navy. He believed that the main causes of constipation were the increased use of refined sugar in diets and the removal of practically all bran from flour during refining. Constipation may be either spastic or nonspastic. Part of the magic of bran is that whether or not your constipation is considered to be spastic, a diet including bran, fresh fruits and vegetables will correct it. Bran is not an irritant.

Another part of the magic of bran is that it has proven very useful in the treatment of diverticulosis (weak areas of the large bowel that have formed pouches extending from the surface of the bowel and open to infection from within the bowel). When these become infected the condition is called diverticulitis. Since this more often involves the left side of the large bowel than the right side, it is sometimes called left-side appendicitis, although it has nothing whatever to do with the appendix.

It has been my experience that the use of bran in the Revitalization Cocktail, as described above, and the combination of the high-protein, low-fat low-sugar diet has been very effective in preventing inflammation in these weakened pouch areas of the large bowel. Of course, if infection develops, your physician will advise you, since surgery may sometimes be required.

Please be sure to drink large quantities of hard water (bottled mineral water) each day. This will be of enormous importance in improving the function of your bowel as well as in providing important minerals for all body functions. The more water you drink, the better it will be for the consistency of your bowel movements. A gallon a day will not be too much, and the result will be softer and larger stools.

Contrasting Effects of Types of Foods

In terms of digestion and bowel action, nothing is superior to bran combined with fresh fruits and vegetables. Again, I must caution you against the supermarket types of breakfast cereals, even those stated to contain bran. There is usually a large amount of sugar in these products, and you should void sugar altogether, wherever possible. Your body does not require refined sugar. Remember that 58 percent of the protein you eat and 10 percent of the fat will be converted into sugar in your body, and *that* sugar is healthful. Indeed, your brain cannot function properly without the energy sugar provides. However, *healthful sugar* is *not the type* found in candy, jams, jellies and supermarket cereals, but the *complex type of carbohydrates* in fruits and in other natural foods. As much as you can, stay away from candy, cookies, cake and white bread. Even some of the darker breads are merely treated with a coloring to make them look dark, whereas they are actually simply white bread. Foods with such high-level sugar content containing no fiber, will not be helpful to your intestinal tract and will definitely be harmful to your entire body.

Some writers have reported that if you take a large quantity of bran in your diet, this bran may combine with certain minerals so that the body cannot absorb these important metals. I do not think that this is a serious consideration for you in my program, especially since you will be taking a high potency vitamin-mineral compound each day. For that matter, you will be getting minerals from other sources as well, if you eat properly.

You may also eat dried fruits to assist you in having good bowel movements. Prunes have an excellent reputation for such action. Since each of us is unique, you will have to determine for yourself just how much bran you can take without excessive flatulence or diarrhea. You will have to make the same determination for the best amount of fruits and vegetables, especially prunes, that you can eat. Do not be impatient. Usually, the excess gas (or gas and diarrhea) does not last more than a few weeks before soft, well-formed stools are passed. However, I must once again emphasize that we are each entirely unique, so you must determine your requirements for yourself.

You have noticed that I add sunflower seeds to the skimmed milk cottage cheese at breakfast, and take such seeds in large quantities at that time. Sunflower seeds contain pectin, and pectin is an important dietary fiber. Not only that, there is some evidence that pectin helps (at least in animal experiments) in ridding the body of undesirable additives. I have read one report by Dr. Fisher, Chairman of the Department of Nutrition at Rutgers University, indicating that pectin "limits the amount of cholesterol the body can absorb." Sunflower seeds produce and provide not only a bran-type effect, but provide pectin (with its reported other benefits), large amounts of iron and potassium and are a high-protein food. If you wish to add soybeans to the sunflower seeds, you have a perfect protein combination, and that is exactly what we have done in the Revitalization Cocktail.

Sunflower seeds also contain the very important linoleic acid, the most important of the essential fatty acids. They even contain their own remedy for oxidation of the unsaturated fats in the form of vitamin E. So, let us not forget the sunflower seeds in the revitalization program.

Bowel Infection and Its Control

I have already told you about the importance of bran as it relates to diverticulosis and diverticulitis. A bowel that empties itself efficiently is more likely to be a healthier one than the one that accumulates large quantities of stool before defecation. I have seen patients who went without a bowel movement for seven or eight days and finally came to me in such a serious condition that it was necessary for me to actually dig out the stool manually with a local anesthesic to protect the muscles around the outlet of the rectum and avoid tearing the lining. If you follow the program I have been describing to this point, if you take adequate quantities of bran and the other bran containing foods, if you eat the revitalization diet and drink the Revitalization Cocktail, you will have brought this type of problem under control. It just will not occur. Your bowel movements will be formed and soft and they will be of much greater quantity than you have experienced before. You will, perhaps for the first time, come very close to actually emptying your bowel each time you go to stool. This is important in removing toxic products from the bowel itself as well as emptying the stool that might otherwise cause pressure against the lining and even infection in outpouching areas, as in diverticulosis.

††*The Story of David L.*

Let me tell you the story of one of my patients, David L., who learned how to control bowel infection and avoided surgery. He had had diverticulosis for many years, was in his early sixties and had been advised that he would probably need surgery one day since he was always constipated and always complaining of pain in the left lower section of his abdomen. Severe pain, tenderness and other evidences of infection in this area, combined with diverticuli, seemed to indicate diverticulitis and require prompt surgery.

He came to me with the hope that I could offer him some treatment for his problem and perhaps avoid surgery. I put him on the entire revitalization program, particularly advising him of the importance of bran, fresh fruits and vegetables and sunflower seeds. I also told him that he could try dried fruits as well, but should not overdo them since we were not looking for a laxative action, but rather for normal, formed, soft stools, passed regularly each morning.

David followed my instructions carefully and happily reported, one month later, that he had excellent bowel movements "every day," and sometimes "twice a day," and "never felt better." He no longer had the tenderness in the lower left section of the abdomen and felt much better in every way. One year later, he returned for a check-up examination, and it was obvious that he not only had revitalized his bowel function, but had renewed his entire body. He looked younger, acted younger, had lost twenty-four pounds and had no complaints whatsoever.

Bran—The High-Fat Diet and Cancer

Many years ago, I published a paper in the *American Journal of Proctology* relating to bran and cancer in Africa. The authority on this subject is Dr. Dennis Burkitt, who has written extensively on the contrast between the natives of rural Africa, who are practically free of cancer and other diseases of the large bowel, and the people of the United States, where such cancer kills almost as many as lung cancer does.

Dr. Burkitt concluded that the cancer-causing agent that may be in the intestinal tract (if there is such an agent) is rapidly eliminated from the colon by the high-fiber diet of the rural African. He stated that the African stool is made up largely of water and fiber and is about four times as large as that in the well-developed Western countries.

There is evidence rapidly developing in the United States that the high-fat diet so common in our country may be related to the development of cancer of the large bowel. One important researcher in cancer speaks of the mushrooming of hamburger stands throughout the United States as the great American "tragedy," based upon this possible relationship between high-fat, high-beef diets and cancer of the bowel.

There have even been reports connecting cancer of the bowel with excessive beer-drinking in certain parts of the United States. Please understand that these are presently opinions of various researchers and that I am not stating that cancer of the bowel is necessarily the direct result of any of these factors. However, they are highly suspect, and if you follow the revitalization diet you will eliminate all of these factors. Without any doubt, you are well-advised to take high levels of bran as described, avoid beef and hamburgers and eat a high-quality ocean fish (or poultry if you prefer to replace fish at times with another high-grade protein product) to reduce the possibility of developing cancer of the colon.

Avoiding or Controlling Hemorrhoids

I have seen hundreds, if not thousands, of patients during the past forty years of practice in proctology, who could have avoided or at least controlled hemorrhoids by the type of diet I have just described. Regrettably, relatively few followed my instructions as they relate to diet, and many preferred surgical removal of the hemorrhoids.

My practice has been to advise patients on the importance of diet, whether or not surgery was required. This is important, since hemorrhoids are simply varicose veins in the rectum and can return in the form of other dilated veins in the rectum if the patient does not follow a proper diet and have regular, easy bowel movements without straining.

If the hemorrhoids are small enough, I usually try injection treatment with a sclerosing agent to shrink the varicose veins. This is very effective in many cases if the patient is seen early enough. Nevertheless, the best way to avoid or control the development of hemorrhoids, is to start the revitalization program before they develop or in their early stages. Most important, of course, is the proper use of bran, fresh fruits and vegetables and the avoidance of straining at stool. Straining at stool can even cause the blood pressure to rise, and if there are weakened blood vessels in the brain, the result may be a stroke during bowel movement. So you will be avoiding or controlling more than hemorrhoids if you follow the revitalization program.

††*How Sarah T. Escaped Pile Surgery*

This is an interesting case of a relatively young woman, in her early thirties. Sarah T., who was very overweight, lived a sedentary life as a housewife and ate the worst possible diet. She was bleeding from the rectum and fearful that she had cancer. I examined the area carefully, and did a sigmoidoscopy to be certain there was no source of bleeding higher in the bowel in addition to the hemorrhoids that I found near the outlet. I then referred her for a careful X-ray study of the bowel, and the report came back negative in every way.

Sarah told me that her hemorrhoids protruded with every bowel movement, and that her stool was small and hard. She often went as long as three days without a bowel movement and then had to take enemas. Her habit was to use soap-sud enemas. I told her that I was opposed to soap-sud enemas, since they acted by irritating the bowel lining. Sarah stopped them at once. I advised her that if she did need an enema she was to use plain warm water or a bulb syringe that would hold at least six ounces of mineral oil. Squeezing the bulb syringe once the lubricated tip is inserted into the lower end of the rectum, would fill the bowel with mineral oil, and the stool would slide out easily.

However, I advised Sarah T. that the best approach was the proper use of nutrition. The instructions I gave her are now well known to you from your three consultations. I asked her to try nutrition alone, but if the bleeding continued, I suggested we might try the injection of the sclerosing solutions as a first step. These are painless injections, by the way. Sarah returned for examination one month later, and was already on her way toward a slim, svelte figure. She still had bleeding from the rectum, but much less than before. We decided that we would not use the injection treatment, but would wait another month or two since she was making excellent progress with relatively easy, formed soft stools. The bran and the other factors in the Revitalization Cocktail had begun their effective cleansing action of the large bowel. She did not return until three months later. At that time, she had a totally new, youthful appearance, both in her face and figure, and happily advised me that the bleeding had stopped altogether. The examination revealed that the hemorrhoids had shrunk to a very small size and no treatment was necessary.

††*Lessons You Have Learned*

1. **Take your Revitalization Cocktail regularly every morning, and add sunflower seeds to the skimmed-milk cottage cheese at breakast.**
2. **Increase the amount of bran gradually until you are having soft, easy, large bowel movements. The increase in bran**

should be taken as additional tablespoonful with lunch or dinner as well as the two tablespoonfuls in your Revitalization Cocktail.

3. Follow the total revitalization diet, and avoid high-fat foods such as steak and hamburger. Substitute ocean fish as your best protein source. If ocean fish is not readily available or if you want variety, chicken or turkey would be fine. If you eat duck, cut away the heavy layer of fat under the skin and do not eat the skin.
4. You must stay on a high-protein, low-fat, low-sugar diet. Fresh fruits and vegetables should be included in your diet every day.

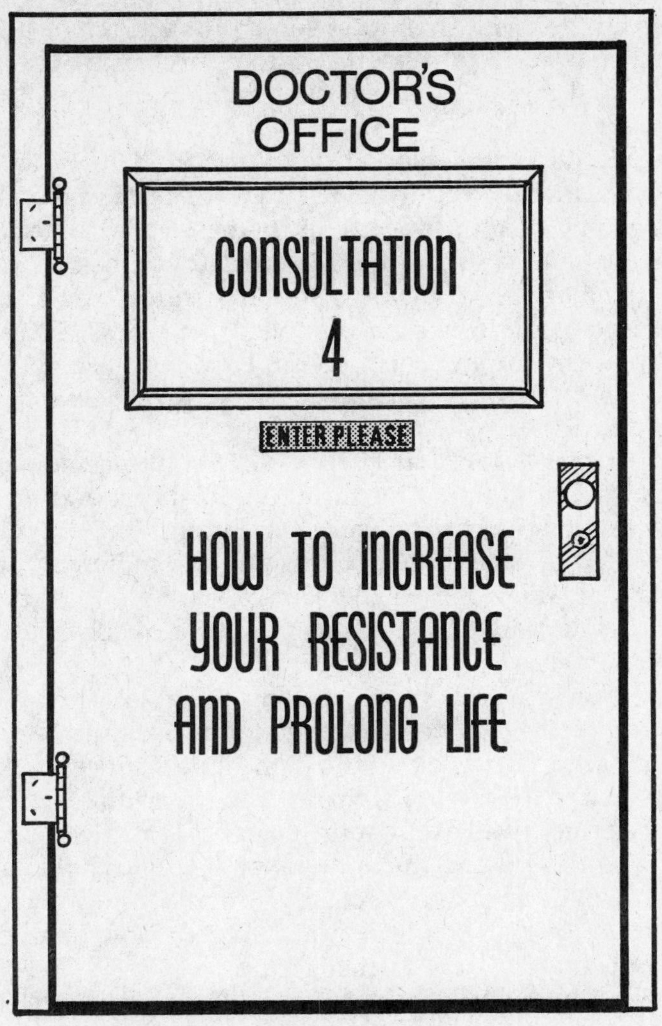

Vitamins for Prevention and Disease Control

Here we are for our fourth consultation. By this time, I am certain that you are fully aware of the tremendous importance of vitamins and minerals for the prevention and control of disease. This is not to say that even the optimal doses of vitamins and minerals will be sufficient by themselves to prevent and control disease. However, since most of us do not eat properly and since most diets are deficient in at least some of the vitamins and minerals (practically all diets are deficient in terms of the optimal level of vitamins and minerals), I have suggested that you supplement your diet.

This becomes particularly important in the Revitalization Program since most of you will be on the half-portion diet in order to reduce excess weight. Indeed, for the best possible health, you should avoid overeating. Your Revitalization Cocktail contains many of the important vitamins for prevention and control of disease, insofar as our present knowledge permits. It also contains some of the important minerals. However, a high potency vitamin-mineral tablet or capsule should also become a part of your daily routine.

It is my impression that vitamin C, vitamin E and selenium are most important for the health and your heart and arteries. I have suggested appropriate amounts throughout the previous consultations. These are the vitamins and the mineral that aid in preventing oxidation of free radicals in your blood stream and tissues. It is this oxidation that seems to be a major factor in the aging of our tissues.

I have advised you, in a previous consultation and in the introduction to this book, of the tremendous importance of maintaining your immune system at the highest possible level. There is a constant battle going on between your immune system and infectious agents such as bacteria and viruses. There is also a continuing battle between the immune system and those cells that tend toward mutation and cancer formation. Immunology is assuming greater and greater importance in medicine, in all phases, not only in the prevention of malignancy.

There is a universally accepted theory that the body forms a certain number of cancer cells each day. If a person's immune system is not functioning adequately, not producing a sufficient number of T-lymphocytes to fight these invasive and potential killer cells, the cancer will progress, and unless that person responds to surgery, radiation and/or chemotherapy, he will die. That is why it is so important that you maintain the best possible health by providing the important nutrients for each cell of your body. By feeding your cells properly, the tissues that are composed of those cells and the organs composed of those tissues will all function to their best advantage—to your best advantage in terms of staying alive, preventing aging and even, in many cases, restoring same degree of youth. Our objective in these consultations is to provide this type of assistance to every cell of your body so that we may revitalize and strengthen every cell, every tissue and every organ of your body-mind.

I reviewed for you, during our second consultation, some important data regarding the "magic" minerals, the gift of the sea, and the particular importance of vitamins for long life. I have also told you about selenium. If you have forgotten any of this discussion, please return to our second consultation and review those sections. It is most important that you understand and apply everything I have told you so that you will indeed increase your resistance and prolong life. Remember that prevention is better than cure, and there may even be the possibility that vitamin in large dosage (10 grams or more per day) and an analog of vitamin A now under study by the National Cancer Institute may even prevent cancer of many of the important organs of your body.

How Arthur L. Reversed the "Incurable"

This patient, 63 years of age, was under my care for the treatment of a colon problem. During this time, he asked my impression of a mole in his armpit. The mole was very black in color, and I suggested that he consult a dermatologist at once, since some moles do carry within themselves a degree of malignancy that is very serious. Please do not be alarmed if you have brown or even black pigmented moles on your body. Practically everyone has a moderate number of such moles and they are usually completely benign. However, I suspected the potential for malignancy in this mole and referred him to a dermatologist of his choice.

He promptly followed my advice, consulted a dermatologist and was told that it would be best for him to have the mole completely removed, possibly including the lymph glands that drain that area into the armpit. The patient was very much alarmed and decided to consult a cancer specialist (an oncologist).

He did so, and the opinion was confirmed as to the need for prompt and radical surgery. When he returned to me with these opinions, he felt that he was on the verge of death from cancer. I told him that he had consulted the proper physicians and that he should proceed at once and follow their advice. Arthur became terribly depressed and felt that he would rather die than undergo extensive surgery, possible chemotherapy and radiation, with all the illness that such therapy produces, despite its frequently very fine results.

Despite the fact that Arthur L. was a very intelligent man, he refused to follow the instructions given to him and said that there was one part of the world that he had not yet seen, and he wanted to do that before undergoing potentially dangerous surgery. He wanted to visit the Orient, especially Japan, China and India. I told him that every day that he waited increased the chance of further spread and that the condition might then become totally and irrevocably incurable.

Since he refused to listen, I advised him to take with him a large supply of Vitamin C tablets (500 mg. per tablet) and a large supply of vitamin A (10,000 units per capsule). I suggested that he might have some success in postponing the evil day during his tour of the Orient by taking 10 grams of vitamin C each day, divided in three relatively equal doses after each meal, taking one or two of the vitamin A capsules each day and staying on the Revitalization Program that I had previously provided for him when he began treatment of his colon problem.

At that time, I had no idea that he planned to stay away for three months, but certainly knew that no matter what I might say beyond what I had already advised, he would not be put off from seeing "as much of the world as possible" before he died.

When he returned, he promptly went into the hospital under the care of the oncologist. The black mole was removed, as were the lymph glands in his armpit. After a relatively brief stay in the hospital, he telephoned me one day to tell me that his surgeon had advised him that he did not need any radiation or chemotherapy. The surgeon had found no malignant tissue in the lymph glands, and had completely removed the malignant mole (it was indeed malignant). His joy was evident in his voice, and his gratitude was expressed in the warmest words, for he generously attributed the control of "the incurable" to my advice. I told him that perhaps it was the result of his strong religious belief, for a great teacher of Judaism and Christianity had once said, "Thy faith will make thee whole." Certainly, I did not wish to take credit for the control of so malignant a disease by nutrition alone.

I believe that Arthur L. was very fortunate, but I urge any of you who are advised to have appropriate surgery for cancer to proceed at once and not depend upon either faith or nutrition to reverse an obviously malignant process.

To further stress this point, I want you to know that if I had a comparable condition, I would have immediate surgery, even though I have naturally been on my own Revitalization Plan and formulas for many years. If time confirms the potential for prevention of a cancer by a vitamin A analog (now under investigation at the National Cancer Institute in Bethesda, Maryland) and the prolongation of life by stimulation of the immune system by Vitamin C in large dosage (as reported by Drs. Cameron and Pauling in Scotland), then we may be able to speak of prevention of certain types of cancer and, possibly, even control. The mainstays will remain, in my opinion, once a diagnosis is established, in the hands of the surgeon, the immunologist, the chemotherapist and the radiation therapist.

Soybean Protein and the Revitalization Cocktail

You will remember that one ingredient of the Revitalization Cocktail is a heaping tablespoonful of lecithin. Lecithin comes from the important soybean. Although cholesterol is essential for your life, your body produces a sufficient amount, and you should not add to it by taking cholesterol or saturated fats in your diet. The high-protein, low-fat, low-sugar diet of the Revitalization Plan will not add to the cholesterol level of your blood stream.

It would seem that one of the best solutions to the cholesterol problem, since cholesterol is deposited in the linings of the arteries and is a major cause of heart attacks and other blood vessel disorders, is to add a large amount of lecithin to your diet. Lecithin acts as an emulsifying agent. This means that if you have a sufficient amount of lecithin in your diet, and therefore in your blood stream, it will help dissolve such cholesterol deposits. We have already spoken of the reports by Dr. L. M. Morrison that showed that about one ounce of lecithin each day for three months will substantially lower cholesterol levels in the blood stream. If you take a sufficient amount of lipotropic factors such as choline, inositol and methionine, these nutrients will assist the body in forming its own lecithin. However, I must stress the importance of the heaping tablespoonful of lecithin in your Revitalization Cocktail for the prevention of cardiovascular disease.

Vitamin B^5 is very important, since it helps in the formation of lecithin. I also suggest magnesium, since this mineral acts in conjunction with vitamin B^6 to reconstitute lecithin after it has been broken down during digestion. As for choline, lecithin is an excellent source. Besides soybeans, there are other excellent sources of the important polyunsaturated linoleic acid. Lecithin itself is available in all health food stores, while other sources are wheat germ (which you are using in your Revitalization Cocktail) and seeds such as sunflower seeds (an important part of your morning breakfast with skimmed milk cottage cheese). I have seen an occasional patient, and internists have seen many more, who have complained of severe headache, sometimes with vomiting, abdominal discomfort and sometimes even numbness in the back after eating Chinese food. They have wondered if this was due to the soybean, and the answer is no. Soybeans do not cause this condition; it is caused by the monosodium glutamate (MSG) used as a flavor enhancer in the preparation of Chinese dishes.

††How Charles X. Achieved New Youth and Sexual Potency

Charles X. was in his late fifties when he first consulted me for hemorrhoids. I removed the hemorrhoids since they were large, protruding and bleeding actively. At the same time, I put him on the Revitalization Cocktail and the other supplements as described for the Revitalization Plan.

During the course of his post-operative treatment, Charles told me that he was impotent and felt that life was really "not worth living." I advised him at that time—about twelve years before writing these consultations—that sexual potency was a matter of the balance between the male hormone (testosterone) and the female hormone (estradiol). What he needed, in my opinion, was the male hormone, as well as the appropriate nutrients in the Revitalization Cocktail and in the Revitalization Plan.

Fortunately Charles X. was not overweight, liked to exercise regularly and did so each morning through "setting up exercises," as well as by playing tennis, golf and bowling. I suggested that he consult an endocrinologist, but he said that he had already consulted several and had been told that it was "all in the mind," and that "he really needed a psychiatrist." He asked me if I would please give him the necessary hormone injections, and I agreed to do so. I told Charles that he would need a large dosage every two weeks, and that once he started on this program of improving hormone levels, he would have to stay with it indefinitely to maintain and retain the new potency and its generalized effect in terms of new youth.

Within a few months after beginning the hormone treatment and the Revitalization Program, Charles X. became sexually active once again, had no difficulty with erection and began to show many signs of reversal of aging.

At the time of this writing, April 1977, there is a report by Dr. Gerald B. Phillips of Columbia University, New York, that male hormone, by injection, may prevent heart attacks in older men. He stated that it is a matter of balance between the female hormone, estradiol, and the male hormone, testosterone. I pointed this out in one of my books, *Doctor Cantor's Longevity Diet*, published by Parker Publishing in 1967. If you will look at page 203 of that book you will find the total picture I describe for longevity, age reversal, revitalization, including reversal of aging of the heart and arteries, with lowering of blood cholesterol. Dr. Phillips believes that the hormones are directly responsible (reduction in the male hormone level), for the heart attacks in older men acting through the secondary factors of a high cholesterol level, fats, sugar and insulin in the blood.

Whatever the mechanism, we should pay more attention to our hormone levels. The all-powerful endocrine glands and their hormones offer the major keys to age reversal and revitalization. But—and this is the big but—your endocrine glands cannot function properly unless you provide them with the essential nutrients, vitamins, minerals and so forth. The ultimate answer, then, is in the molecules that make up the cells, and those molecules must be literally fed and bathed by an optimal level of nutrients.

My Revitalization Cocktail and my Revitalization Plan will provide the best possible sustenance for those cells at the molecular level. Cells that are well fed at that level will function at their optimal capacity. This, in turn, means that the tissues made up of those cells and the organs made up of those tissues will function to their best capacity.

Effect of Vitamins in Mega Dosage

Throughout these consultations, I have spoken of the use of vitamins in optimal level amounts. I did not speak of "mega dosage," only because I believe that we must individualize the amount for each person, depending upon their unique needs and their unique capacity for absorption and utilization of vitamins.

Naturally, if your physician believes in the use of mega dosage, follow his advice. No one can possibly know your individual needs better than the physician who is caring for you. Some of the levels that I advise, such as those for vitamin C, go beyond the ordinary mega dosage simply because there is excellent evidence that this vitamin may be helpful in stimulating the immune system. You already know the enormous importance of this. For those who cannot tolerate as much as 10 grams daily, the amount taken should obviously be reduced. As for vitamin E, the usual mega dosage recommended is exactly the amount that I have been advising for the Revitalization Cocktail, 800 I.U. per day.

Vitamin C can cause excessive passage of gas from the bowel and possibly diarrhea. If so, and if this is offensive to you, reduce the amount accordingly. Personally, I have found that for myself and for those of my patients who have stayed with the level I have recommended, this is a rarely troublesome development, and usually stops entirely after a few weeks or months. Sometimes, there is some irritation of the urinary passage, in which case you would be well advised to find a combination of half ascorbic acid and half sodium ascorbate. Both forms are vitamin C, regardless of the chemical formula.

I do not know of any toxic evidence reported for vitamin E. The mega level of vitamin A recommended goes up to 200,000 I.U. This is not a toxic level in the average adult but should not be continued for very long. Consult your physician. I prefer that you stay at a level no more than 35,000 I.U. each day. Some physicians recommend gradually increasing the amount of the various vitamins over a period of time. You may try this, if you wish, but I have found in my personal life and in my practice that the levels already suggested during these consultations are quite safe for adults, and seem to be an optimal dosage for the average person.

††*How Roy V. Restored Health and Energy*

Roy V. was a harassed advertising executive. His work placed him under great stress, because he handled important accounts. Every lunch was a business lunch and involved several potent cocktails as well as wines and very rich French food. Roy truly believed that the French cuisine was the best in the world. Perhaps he is right in terms of taste, but he is certainly wrong in terms of the butter content in most French dishes. Roy was eating a very high-fat, high-sugar diet, enormously high in calories as well and filled with the empty calories of alcohol. When I saw Roy, it was for the treatment of colitis. He also needed the assistance, I felt, of a good psychologist or psychiatrist, as well as someone who specialized in restoring an alcoholic to normal.

I suggested, as gently as I could, that his diet, the alcoholism, and the stress of his way of life all conspired to destroy his health and reduce his energy bank. He laughed and said, "I agree with you, but I am fifty-four years of age, making a very fine income, doing a good job and it is too late for me to change." My response was that if he did not change he had relatively little time left to live. More important, whatever time he had left, could scarcely be appreciated by anyone in his condition.

Despite his initial denial, he did want to live and agreed to place himself on the Revitalization Formula and the Revitalization Plan. I suggested that he would probably find good company in Alcoholics Anonymous, and he even agreed to attend their meetings. Obviously, Roy's drive for survival was as great as his drive for self-destruction. It is curious how so many of us dance about the golden calf and, when it is too late, find that our life is gone and we have never noticed the blue sky, the green trees or even smelled the flowers.

Alcoholics Anonymous was most successful with my patient. Without that organization, the treatment of his colitis and the restoration of his health and energy would probably have been a failure. Roy V. followed my instructions closely as they related to the teachings of this book, gave up French food and to this day, ten years later, is still on the half-portion diet. I suggested that he take long walks each day, preferably in Connecticut, his home area, rather than in New York, because the air was more breathable and less dangerous. During these long walks, he was to repeat to himself, "Younger and younger, healthier and healthier, happier and happier." These long walks, combined with the Revitalization Cocktail and the miracle of "drying out" from alcohol, restored both health and energy to this fine man. His skin took on the glow of youth, his step was now bouncy and young and his energy was practically unlimited. To use his own words, "I am a better man now in business and at home than I ever was before."

The Magic of Selenium

I have already told you about selenium and its importance as an anti-oxidant. It ranks with vitamin C and vitamin E in that respect and is therefore very important in the prevention of aging and even in the restoration of youth. Selenium is now available in combination with vitamin C in health food stores. I do not know if it can be obtained in pharmacies, but it seems to be used extensively in animal feed. It is curious how animals raised for market often receive better care and better food than people.

I have already told you that onions contain selenium, and I personally like to eat the whole raw onion, almost as if it were an apple. It is also found in organ meats, and if you wish to take liver as an occasional substitute for fish and poultry, I have no objection. You will also find selenium in fruits and vegetables, cereals and nuts. The Revitalization Plan includes selenium as well as the other anti-oxidants.

††*How a Doctor Learned an Important Lesson*

Doctors learn very little about nutrition in medical school. When I graduated medical school, so many years ago that I don't like to think about it, I had learned absolutely nothing about nutrition. All the doctors that I knew were overweight with rare exception, they were overworked and usually died relatively early from a "coronary." Cardiovascular disease was and is very common among physicians. Doctors really obtain very little exercise, work hard, are dedicated to their profession, and completely ignore their own health. It is always "do as I say and not as I do."

A very good physician friend of mine in his mid-forties suffered a mild stroke. When he recovered from the stroke, he asked if I would have lunch with him. During the luncheon, he said, "I have been sending you patients for a long time for surgery and I know—from them—that you have placed many of them on a proper diet, much to their benefit." He then went on to ask if I would do the same for him.

I asked the doctor about his general health. He then stated the facts as he saw them, "I have had a stroke, as you know, and my blood pressure remains high despite all medications. I am overweight, as you can see. I know that if I don't get rid of this weight and restore some flexibility to my arteries, I will have a major stroke or a coronary, and that will be that." I told him that I would be very happy to tell him about my plan for revitalization and restoration of youth to aging arteries and heart, but I could make no promises. I then went on to say, "I know that you see a great many patients each day as an internist, that you work long, hard hours and that you must be under continuous stress. Would you be willing to cut your practice by one-third, in terms of time, and learn to relax?" He was willing to do anything I said, because he realized that survival was indeed more important than the accumulation of a large practice.

He followed the Revitalization Plan very closely and within three months showed an improvement in the level of his blood pressure, a loss of weight, and the restoration of a more youthful figure and appearance. He continued on this plan, even to this day, and as of this writing seems to be in perfect health, excellent spirits and looks very well indeed.

Food for the Mind—Even the Depressed Mind

When you are following the Revitalization Plan, you will be providing the best possible food for the nervous system as well as for the rest of your body. This is what I mean by proper food for the mind. It is really proper nutrition for the mind-body. The central nervous system cannot function adequately unless it is provided with adequate nutrients, and is not handicapped by a toxic internal or external environment.

The internal environment consists partly of the nutrients supplied by your diet and partly by the ideas in your mind. Everything that has ever happened to you, from the beginning of your time on Earth, is permanently recorded in your mind. Your day-to-day problems, combined with the anxieties of even the distant past, can become overwhelming. You may become depressed and sometimes even suicidal to the extent that you may follow self-destructive practices.

††*The Case of Barbara A.*

One of my young patients, Barbara A., a very well-educated professor of psychology, teaching in a major university, suffered bouts of severe depression. This was accompanied by nausea, vomiting at times and an overactive large bowel. It was because of these symptoms that she consulted me.

I told her that she might be well advised, since her depressions were very severe, to consult another psychologist or a psychiatrist. Barbara said that she had been under the care of a psychiatrist, but was so depressed at times that she could not eat at all, while at other times, she ate too much, even of foods she knew were self-destructive. She would eat an entire box of chocolates at one time, *realizing* at the time that what she was doing was reverting to her childhood, to the candy pacifier.

I told her that the relationship between her gastrointestinal tract and her central nervous system must be very obvious to her in relation to her understanding of psychosomatic medicine. Certainly, she had to be aware that the gastrointestinal tract is a creature of the mind. The relationship is very close, and often the best treatment for a disturbed gastrointestinal tract is treatment of the emotional problems. Her major emotional problem was that she was not advancing rapidly in her department and was fearful that she might not obtain tenure. I asked her if it was worthwhile dying to become tenured. She looked at me as if I were mad and responded, "Not at all."

I pointed out that if she continued along her present path, destroying her emotional balance as well as her body, she was certainly headed toward self-destruction, to the point of death. I suggested that she lower her sights as far as advancement toward a permanent professorship and begin thinking in terms of survival—one day at a time. I pointed out that none of us can live more than one day at a time, indeed only one heartbeat at a time. Barbara was a religious girl, a Protestant, and I reminded her that a great teacher, Jesus, had once said, "Sufficient unto the day the evils thereof." No one could live more than one day at a time, and there were certainly sufficient problems during that day without worrying about past failures or future demands. We all have problems and can only solve them from moment to moment, from day to day.

Meanwhile, I suggested that she learn to give her full attention to the present moment so that she would no longer be constantly harassed by the fears of the future and the problems of the past. I taught her how to relax her entire body and suggested that she practice this relaxation technique each evening before going to sleep and each morning when she awoke. She was also to take long walks, even in bad weather, and while walking she was to occupy her brain with the words "Healthier and healthier, younger and younger, healthier and healthier, younger and younger," with each step. She was to allow no other words to enter her mind. While she was repeating this, she was to concentrate upon the sights, the sounds, and the smells around her. In other words, I was teaching her how to live *now*.

Naturally, I also advised her of the importance of proper nutrition in terms of the Revitalization Plan. She enjoyed the Revitalization Formula, followed the plan completely and in very short order was able to give up her psychiatrist and live a relatively normal life. One year later, she had transferred to another university, and her new personality and attitude toward life made her very popular with the faculty. Barbara soon became an important figure within the university faculty and attained tenure.

How to Think Young

What I was doing with Barbara A. was teaching her how to think young and think healthy, and you can do the same. First, you should learn to relax. I suggest that while reading this, you should lie down flat on your back. Now, talk to your toes and tell them to relax, tell your feet to relax, your ankles, your legs, your knees, your thighs, your buttocks. Go on to tell your abdomen, your chest, your shoulders, your arms, your elbows, your forearms, your wrists and your hands to relax. Now we come to the most important areas for relaxation. Tell your neck to relax, your mouth, your nose, your cheeks, your eyes, your forehead and your scalp.

You may reverse this procedure if you wish, and start with the top of your head. The most important areas to relax are around the eyes, the forehead and the muscles around the mouth. When these muscles are relaxed, all the others will relax more readily. People who frown constantly or purse their lips, are tightening the muscles of the forehead, the muscles around the eyes and the muscles of the mouth. It is important to relax these muscles, so pay special attention to that area.

Now that you are completely relaxed, let yourself go into an even deeper state of relaxation by quieting your mind. The best way to do that is to repeat to yourself, "Younger and younger, younger and younger, younger and younger." When you do, you will be programming your mind with youth and neutralizing the aging that results from tight, stress-controlled muscles. It is important to do this as often as possible, certainly in the morning when you wake and at night before you go to sleep.

How to Overcome Problems of the Past and Fear of the Future

When you are fully relaxed, when you are walking and when you are working, as often as you possibly can, leave the anxieties of the past behind and overcome the fear of the future by concentrating your full attention on what is going on about you. If you are giving full attention, truly and completely, to the present moment, the past and future cease to bedevil the mind. If you still find anxieties rising to a conscious level, you must then practice Mantra meditation.

The Mantra is a series of words or syllables, originally in Sanskrit or other ancient languages, which has been used for meditation to quiet the mind for thousands of years, particularly in Eastern cultures. You may use the Mantra type of meditation while relaxed or even while at work if you want to push troubling thoughts out of your mind. Repeat what is considered to be the universal sound of the world—*Om*. Say this over and over again to yourself, drawing out the words as if you were saying *Aum* rather than *Om*. This will give you the sound of the ancient Mantra. This type of repetition of a word that has a universal meaning, totally unrelated to your anxieties, will help to quiet your mind. When it is fully quiet, you should then go on to say, "Younger and younger, younger and younger, healthier and healthier, healthier and healthier." You will thus be re-programming your now quiet mind with a positive, healthful, youth-restoring phrase. In this fashion, you will be well on your way toward overcoming the problems of the past and the fears of the future.

††*Your Prescriptions for Today . . .*

1. Relax daily, at least twice, in the morning upon arising and at night before going to sleep. Relax your entire body and mind. Then think young and use the Mantra for youth and revitalization.
2. Be sure to take your vitamins, not only with the Revitalization Cocktail, but with your high potency capsule or tablet. Don't miss a single day.
3. Be sure to take your minerals in terms of the proper foods such as fruits, vegetables, sunflower seeds, onions, sea food, sardines, and so forth.
4. If you are losing sexual potency, consult your physician. You may need to achieve a new hormonal balance.

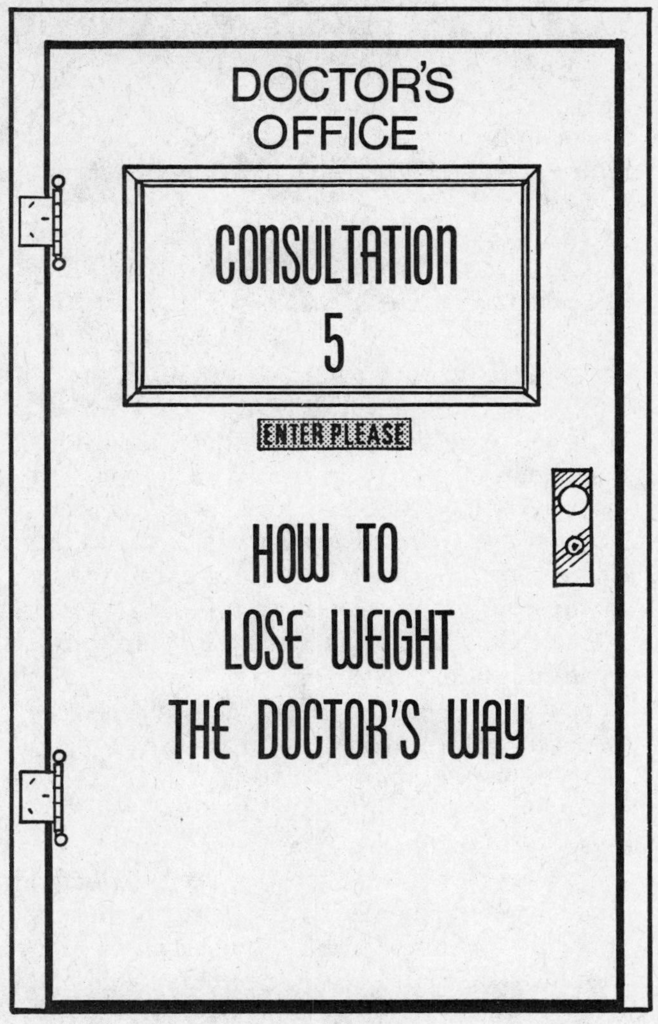

DOCTOR'S
OFFICE
CONSULTATION
5
ENTER PLEASE
HOW TO
LOSE WEIGHT
THE DOCTOR'S WAY

It is a pleasure, once again, to be with you for our fifth consultation. By this time, you have learned a great deal about the significance of the Revitalization Cocktail and the Revitalization Plan. You now know that you can indeed slow aging and restore youth, and you also know how to do it. There is still a great deal more to learn, but if you have clearly understood and begun the application of the first four consultations to your daily life, you are probably already beginning to see results.

You have learned how to relax, how to quiet your mind, how to eat properly, how to control your bowel function, how to improve the health of your heart and arteries and many other important new ways of living for a healthier mind and body. During this consultation we will talk entirely about the question of losing weight.

A Doctor's Formulation for Healthier Heart and Arteries

The health of your heart and arteries determines to a large extent how long you will live. Cardiovascular disease is a major cause of death in practically all civilized countries. Indeed, with the inroads being made by "civilization," and "civilized" foods within the underdeveloped nations, heart and artery disease is now becoming a problem in those countries as well. The proper approach must be through understanding the importance of nutrition and actually applying this understanding in your daily life. You must take your Revitalization Cocktail each morning. If you follow my own formulation for a healthier heart and cleaner arteries, you will also take skimmed milk cottage cheese with a large sprinkling (one or more ounces) of sunflower seeds. The sunflower seeds are very important for many reasons, which I have told you about in a previous consultation.

You will also add to your breakfast the whites of two hard-boiled eggs. Throw away the yolks for they are full of cholesterol. They also contain lecithin, which is important for the control of cholesterol, but you have already had your lecithin "straight" in the Revitalization Cocktail. No need to have the cholesterol itself, since that adds a serious danger to your arteries and heart.

If you wish to complete your breakfast with a decaffeinated coffee, I have no objection. However, once you have given up coffee, you will have no difficulty in staying away from it completely, whether or not it has caffeine in it.

You will, of course, avoid all cola drinks, since they have a high level of caffeine as well. They also contain sugar or a sugar substitute, both of which are dangerous from different points of view. The sugar substitute is now under attack as a potential cause of cancer, and sugars, as you know, are dangerous for your heart and arteries in their own way. You must avoid candy, cake, cookies, saturated fats and starch foods, and you must eliminate naked calories. The naked calories are those found in food that have no nutritional value such as ordinary table sugar, as well as the sugar in the candy and cake category.

Take the "magic" minerals in a supplementary high potency vitamin-mineral capsule or tablet and in natural form in ocean fish, especially the herring family. Even if you do not like fish now, by eating it regularly, you will soon develop a taste for it and will learn to like not only the fish, but the renewed youth and the greater health.

When I started to lose weight, I had the difficulty of a well-trained appetite, demanding food regularly. I learned to control the appetite by drinking my original *Longevity Diet Cocktail* before each meal. That cocktail contained one ounce of safflower oil, and the safflower oil acted as a natural appetite depressant while providing me with what I consider to be the best possible amount of polyunsaturated oil—three ounces each day.

I later found that I could do without the safflower oil in the afternoon and evening as I began to lose weight. The half-portion approach, combined with my recognition of the fact that I really did want to stay alive and avoid premature death from a heart attack, offered a sufficient combination to reduce my appetite and prevent me from eating foods that were self-destructive. Believe me, once you have reached this point in your thinking, in your understanding with the level of information that you now have, you will not miss the excess food that you used to eat. Certainly, you won't miss the excess weight. Your heart will be grateful. It will no longer need to pump an enormous amount of blood through the capillaries (the tiny blood vessels) in the excess fat you formerly carried throughout your body.

I began to practice walking each morning and whenever otherwise possible during the day, especially when I was in a part of the country where the air was breathable and not heavily polluted as it is in the heart of New York and New Jersey as well as in many other parts of the United States and the rest of the world. I began with slow walking and gradually increased the pace as well as the time. You only need twenty or thirty minutes of walking to improve the health of your heart and arteries as well as your general feeling of well being. While walking, I would repeat to myself, "Healthier and healthier, happier and happier, younger and younger." This is the mind-body approach to the Revitalization Program.

During our sixth consultation, I will tell you more about how to loosen stiff joints and aching muscles and about the important Buddha Walk and the Buddha Dance for renewed energy, lung, heart and muscle strength. For the present, however, you need only practice simple walking in the fashion I have just described. This was my formulation, and I lost forty pounds the easy way and in a relatively short time by following this formulation.

††How Husband and Wife Lost a Combined One Hundred Pounds the Easy Way

Good friends, Bob and Eleanor T., observing my loss of weight and the revitalization of my appearance and new youth, asked me if I would tell them how they could lose weight. I advised them that the first step was a careful study by their private physician to make certain they had no serious disorders, especially no serious disease of the heart and arteries. After that, if they wished to talk to me about the problem, I would be pleased to advise them. Bob and Eleanor came to me two weeks later with a report from their cardiologist showing a completely normal heart and artery pattern, with the exception of the tendency toward an elevated blood pressure for both husband and wife. The cardiologist had advised them to lose weight and to return for a reexamination in six months.

I then instructed them on the Revitalization Cocktail, my revitalization breakfast, and the importance of the half-portion method of eating.

Both Bob and Eleanor smoked incessantly, and I told them that unless they gave up cigarette smoking entirely, they were only going part way toward restoration of youth and prevention of aging. I told them of the great danger of lung cancer for cigarette smokers. They did not know that women are now suffering from lung cancer almost as much as men, since larger numbers of women have begun smoking cigarettes. Lung cancer is the major cause of cancer death in men, and most lung cancer patients die within the first six months after diagnosis. Only 7 percent live as long as five years after surgery, radiation and/or chemotherapy. The same statistics would no doubt apply to women.

I pointed out that there was very little value in losing weight if the slender body was then going to be destroyed by cigarette smoking. They found it more difficult to give up cigarettes than they did to give up food, but they recognized the importance of my message and were both sufficiently intelligent and sufficiently motivated to follow instructions carefully. I also advised them on the importance of walking daily; at least twenty or thirty minutes of brisk walking was recommended once they had become accustomed to the technique and repetition of the "better and better, healthier and healthier, younger and younger" formula.

When Bob and Eleanor T. returned to their cardiologist six months later, they had lost a combined one hundred pounds and told him—as they had previously told me—that they had never felt better, that they had greater energy than ever before and that they certainly enjoyed life more.

How to Enjoy Meals

The enjoyment of meals, like the enjoyment of anything else, requires that you give your full attention to what you are doing. While eating, you should not be reading a book or a newspaper. You should be concentrating on the food. You should take small portions into your mouth, not large bulky amounts that extend your cheeks like a chipmunk. You should chew your food slowly, relishing the taste, the flavor and the quality of the food.

When you drink your Revitalization Cocktail, you should sip it relatively slowly. My practice is to eat the cottage cheese with the sunflower seeds a teaspoonful at a time, chewing the cheese and the sunflower seeds thoroughly at the corners of the mouth so that the molars do the job. Enjoy the crunchiness of the sunflower seeds, the taste, the juicy cottage cheese and its taste, and after you have chewed it thoroughly and enjoyed it thoroughly, then swallow a mouthful. This will take time. You cannot gulp your meals down and enjoy them no matter how well prepared the food may be.

Your mind should not be burdened by anxiety while eating. Normally, most of us rush through a meal, whether it is at home or at fast-food counters of the hamburger or fried chicken variety. That food is both self-destructive and relatively dangerous to all parts of the body. It may even have some relationship to cancer formation. Knowing this—just knowing this—should be sufficient to steer you away from all such foods—the foods that contain additives, the foods that are high in fat content, the foods that are simply naked calories like sugar, cake, candy and such, and all the other foods that I have already told you about that act to destroy the body and cause premature aging. How can you possibly enjoy eating such foods now that you know they are a form of suicide every time you eat them?

You cannot enjoy sex with your wife or husband if your mind is elsewhere. In the same way, you cannot enjoy food if your mind is occupied with anxieties. Therefore, to take your mind away from the problems of the past and the fears of the future, your daily business anxieties, that annoying customer or problem that you must solve or pacify before the day is over, keep your mind clear of these problems by substituting the following formula as you chew, "Healthier and healthier, happier and happier, younger and younger—every day in every way." Or, you might prefer, "Healthier and healthier, healthier and healthier, healthier and healthier." Or simply, "Younger and younger, younger and younger, younger and younger." With the repetition of this formula, the complete attention to your food, the total awareness of the taste, quality, texture of the food, and finally—and perhaps above all—the realization that you are in the process of restoring your youth, slowing the aging process and perhaps on the way toward living one hundred years of a happy, healthy life, you will finally—perhaps for the first time—be enjoying your meals.

††*How a Doctor Lost Weight and Regained New Energy the M-B Way*

First, let me explain what I mean by the M-B way. This refers to the mind-body concept. By this time, you know that your mind is in every cell of your body, and whether it is a matter of losing weight, regaining new energy, slowing aging or restoring youth, it all adds up to survival and a longer life for those who do it the mind-body way.

You will notice that I have brought the mind into the picture throughout this entire book. Stress acts through the mind to destroy the body. Stress is the antagonist of the mind-body. The mind-body approach to revitalization will reduce stress. When you reduce stress, the body can then utilize the proper nutrients to rebuild itself, revitalize itself and become younger. So you must always use the mind-body approach in your effort to revitalize and strengthen your mind-body.

A good friend, Frank P., an active surgeon who operated practically every day of the week, had become very obese, eating the worst type of meals in the hospital cafeterias as well as when he entertained friends at home or in restaurants. He always had one or two cocktails before meals and enjoyed the best French wines. Naturally, the cocktails and wines were not available in the hospital cafeterias, but they were freely available in every other place he choose to dine. His heart was beginning to show signs of strain, and he was on the verge of a very high level of hypertension. The possibility of a serious heart and artery disorder had finally broken down his resistance, and he asked for my help. I gave Frank a copy of my *Longevity Diet* book, and he began on that program. After six months, I suggested to him that he replace the Longevity Diet Cocktail (The Cantor Cocktail), with the Revitalization Cocktail formula that I am describing in this set of consultations. And so, for the past years, right up to the present moment (I hope for many years to come), he has been on the Revitalization Cocktail and Plan exactly as you are now studying it. As a surgeon, Frank regrettably knew nothing about psychosomatic medicine and rebelled at first at my concept of the mind-body approach. He thought it rather foolish to be repeating, within his own mind, "Younger and younger, younger and younger, younger and younger," as I had instructed him to do while eating and while taking long walks. Indeed, I suggested to him that since his surgery was now practically automatic and required little thinking, he might very well use this formula to occupy his mind throughout the morning while operating.

Gradually, Frank realized the importance of what I was saying and did exactly that. He was using the M-B approach practically all day long, while eating, in surgery, while walking and before going to sleep. The results were amazing. He lost well over 60 pounds within the first seven months, began to operate even more efficiently than he had in the past, certainly enjoyed his food more since he was now giving it his full attention and had been released from the lethargy effect and the bondage of alcohol. Frank had given up his cocktails and French wines and could now say, "I really don't miss them!"

How to Lose Pounds and Add Years of Living

It is obvious now, that I have been telling you exactly how to lose pounds. When you are overweight, the loss of these extra pounds will reduce the burden on your heart and arteries. Each pound of fat contains miles of tiny capillaries, and the heart must pump blood through each of these tiny vessels. When you reduce the strain on the heart by losing weight, the heart muscle can then revitalize itself and regain its health.

Remember that you are as old as your arteries and that you are as young as your renewed, revitalized arteries when you are well embarked on the Revitalization Program. Finally, remember that you will be as happy as you think you are, and apply the mind-body approach to your thinking. When you do this, you will not only add years of living while you lose excess weight, you will also be adding happiness to those years of living. The reduction of stress when the mind is emptied is tremendous. The mind is the killer, since stress is the killer and stress is a product of the mind.

Learn to set a limit to your desires. You cannot possibly have all the money in the world and there will always be someone who has more than you. You only need enough to provide food, clothing and shelter for yourself and your family. I hesitate to say that you need enough for your retirement, since with current inflation levels and the various other problems relating to the currencies of the world, it would appear that only the multi-millionaires can attain sufficient levels of money for a satisfying retirement. The rest of us will have to do the best we can by simplifying life.

I think that an important mind-body concept is to simplify life right now. If you are living in a large house and your children have already grown and left you, sell the house. If you cannot sell the house and can afford to abandon it, do so. Move into smaller quarters in a climate that will not burden your health or your purse. Again, I recommend that you set a limit to your desires.

When you practice the Revitalization Program, you will be reducing the amount of food you eat, which will automatically reduce the cost of living in terms of your food needs. If you simplify life by getting rid of excess baggage such as a house that you have outlived, expensive car that you really don't need and even the enormous business pressures that you subjected yourself to in order to build your personal business, only then will you be truly living. At that point, your mind-body approach to new youth will begin to show its fullest effect. Released from pressures, without the enormous burdens of your past, most of the stress of that type of living will be gone. It is then that the Revitalization Formula and Revitalization Plan will show the greatest effect. You will become a new person, healthier, happier, younger from day to day.

††*How Bob R. Lost Weight and Found New Arteries*

One final case history before we close this consultation. Bob R. is interesting because he did not follow my advice, although referred by his own physician to me. He nearly lost his life. He was sixty-two years of age and very much overweight, with the beginning of a very serious cardiovascular condition. He had constipation so severe that he could not move his bowels more than once every three or four days, and then he had to take enemas, all of which caused active rectal bleeding.

After careful examination, I found that Bob R. had no serious pathology in the large bowel or the rectum. I suggested that he begin the Revitalization Cocktail, telling him of the importance of bran and the appropriate nutrients to the health of his entire body and especially for the avoidance of constipation at this time. He was a very slow starter and although quite intelligent, seemed bent on suicide.

When I noted the fact that his progress was very slow, I asked Bob whether he preferred to die or wished to live. I put it to him bluntly, in just those words. He said nothing, but seemed subdued. I then went on to say, "If you continue doing as you are doing now and do not follow my instructions, I must assume that you wish to commit suicide. You may do that, if that is what you want. But if you really want to live, if you really want to learn how to enjoy whatever is left of life, you will have to start on my plan of treatment and start on it immediately. Otherwise, you will soon have a serious heart and blood vessel condition, and I doubt that you will live more than a relatively short time afterward. Your family doctor has told you this, your cardiologist has told you this and now I tell you." Bob still did not respond, but merely seemed to shrink further into his chair. I continued, "Think about it, and if you can't make a decision now, come back when you do and let me know."

He did not come back for three months, and I assumed that he had decided to go his own way, come what may. I was wrong. He had given my words serious thought and had come to the conclusion that I was right, that he was indeed committing suicide. He told his wife what I had said, and she came with him at this visit.

It was she who spoke first, "We came to thank you. The problem was mine as much as Bob's. I think—I know—that I was demanding too much of him and that he was overworked. I have enough jewelry for three women, enough fur coats for three and we will have enough to live on if he earns one-third of what he has been earning." Her husband interrupted, "I am not the wealthiest of men, but I do have a fine family, and I do want to stay alive. I did not realize, until you spoke to me bluntly, that I was, indeed, committing suicide. I have been following your instructions, and as you can see, I have lost weight and feel much better. My cardiologist tells me that my heart and arteries are responding well. My blood pressure is down and my most recent electrocardiogram is normal."

They both thanked me, with tears in their eyes, and to the best of my knowledge, they are both well and happy, living in a warmer climate on the West Coast.

The Liquid Protein Diet

This is a controversial diet for rapid weight loss. It is controversial because those who drink the hydrolyzed (enzyme predigested) liquid protein from the fibrous protein collagen of animal tissues, do so more often than not without a doctor's preliminary study and continuing observation. Some such self-starters suffer from various problems that seem to be related to the liquid protein diet, such as constipation, dizziness, bad breath, dry skin and even loss of hair. There may be serious underlying problems, unknown to the dieter, involving one or more organs or systems that would perhaps contraindicate this approach to dealing with obesity.

No one should seriously restrict their diet to a single component drink (protein only) for each meal (with no other food) unless and until they have been carefully monitored and checked out by a competent doctor. They should also be instructed in the mind-body approach to proper motivation during this strenuous dietary regime. Unless they are correctly motivated to remain on a low-calorie, half-portion diet, after they have finished their crash course in weight loss, most will soon regain the former weight level.

The liquid protein concept was developed by Dr. George Blackburn, an associate professor of surgery at Harvard Medical School, as a protein-sparing solution for very sick patients. Note this: it was given intravenously. Such patients then burned the predigested intravenous protein, and this spared the vital protein in the body's life-support organs. Dr. Blackburn later applied this concept to overweight patients who were otherwise healthy, but again note that it was meant to replace lean meat and poultry. These natural foods offer the same protein amino acids as the liquid protein formulas and have the added advantage of allowing the stomach to digest and absorb the protein building blocks (the amino acids) in normal fashion rather than by vein or in predigested form by mouth.

A very important advantage of eating the natural source of high-protein, low-fat food, is that this is the normal way for us to learn to eat properly, with pleasure and in controlled measure. It is unnatural to depend upon an artificially prepared and predigested drink for every meal. The revitalization diet and the total Revitalization Program offers you the natural way to lose weight.

Even more than that, the program's approach to total health of mind and body does much more than simply reduce excess pounds. The mind-body approach—at the same time—restores better health and greater vitality to all cells, tissues and organs of your body. Another product, used in the same way to produce predigested protein drinks, is made from egg albumen. As you now know, the Revitalization Diet includes the whites of two hard-boiled eggs. Again, the natural approach rather than the manufactured product.

The Longevity, Revitalization Diet and Program for Weight Loss

Now, by contrast, let us give further consideration to the natural way—the doctor's way—to lose weight while revitalizing the entire body-mind. The high-protein, low-fat (polyunsaturated), low-sugar, low-starch, caffeine-free diet offered in the Revitalization Program is the royal road to losing those excess pounds. You will lose them permanently, not in an energy-depleting crash-course fashion with possible serious harm to your general health.

If you use a skimmed milk base and add one heaping tablespoonful of soy flour, one heaping tablespoonful of lecithin, one level tablespoonful of brewer's yeast flakes, one ounce of safflower oil and flavor it as you wish with decaffeinated coffee, one of the many natural fruit flavors available in health food stores or, perhaps, carob powder (for its natural chocolate-like taste), your blender will produce a delightful, healthful, weight-reducing drink.

Let this be your total breakfast, if you wish, but also take a high potency vitamin-mineral capsule or tablet. You may make this your lunch as well, if you choose, and save the "big meal" for dinner. That meal will be fish or fowl, preferably ocean fish, chicken or turkey, a large green vegetable salad and lightly cooked (pressure-cooked if possible) vegetables.

To give you some idea of the wonderful protein content of low-fat soy flour, one pound of the soy flour is equal to three dozen eggs, over seven quarts of milk, two pounds of cheese or two-and-one-half pounds of meat! The amount you will put in your drink will be one heaping tablespoonful, unless you are a real heavyweight who is over 250 pounds. Then, you may use two heaping tablespoonfuls of the soy flour.

The base may be an unsweetened fruit juice of your choice, rather than skimmed milk. I like orange juice for my own Revitalization Cocktail, especially since I add five grams of vitamin C to my drink (twice each day for a total of 10 grams). The alkaline soy flour neutralizes the acidity of the vitamin C, another advantage of the Cocktail.

More on Low Fat Soy Powder

Low-fat soy powder is available in health food stores and is not at all expensive in contrast to the liquid protein preparations. The powder is from a vegetable source (the magic soybean) and is a healthful alkaline food that may be helpful in neutralizing the acidity of other foods such as meats and grains. The approximate nutrient analysis of the soy powder (flour) is: protein 50 percent, polyunsaturated oil—6 percent, carbohydrate—11 percent and lecithin—2.3 percent, and it also provides large amounts of phosphorus, iodine, calcium, thiamine, niacin and riboflavin.

If you must eat between meals, try chewing on raw carrots or stalks of celery. You may even have "an apple a day to keep the doctor away." As you know, I like to add still more protein to my breakfast by eating the whites of two hard boiled eggs. I also add cottage cheese, supplemented by sunflower seeds. You may prefer to keep these two items for in-between snacks—but only if you must. If you truly want to lose weight the doctor's way, you will stay with the basic pattern I have already advised for the Revitalization Plan. You will lose weight and regain youth if you do.

My patients have lost an average of 10 to 30 pounds in the very first month. You may lose more or less (there is no hurry!), but be sure to weigh yourself on an accurate scale immediately upon arising and after emptying bowel and bladder each morning. If you add the wheat germ bran to your morning "cocktail," you will have an easy, large bowel movement each morning. This is of enormous importance for your Revitalization Program. Stay with this program after you have lost the unnecessary and self-destructive extra pounds and you will see a new you—younger, healthier and more vigorous than ever.

††*Your Instructions for Today*

1. **Use the M-B formula every day, while eating, before sleeping and even while at work if your time permits.**
2. **When you use the M-B formula, eat slowly, savor each mouthful. You will enjoy your food, and the half-portion will not only be adequate but very satisfying.**
3. **Lose excess weight by following the entire Revitalization Plan. When you lose weight you will add years of living.**
4. **The M-B approach to all of life will give you greater happiness, better health, and longer life. Live each day the M-B way.**

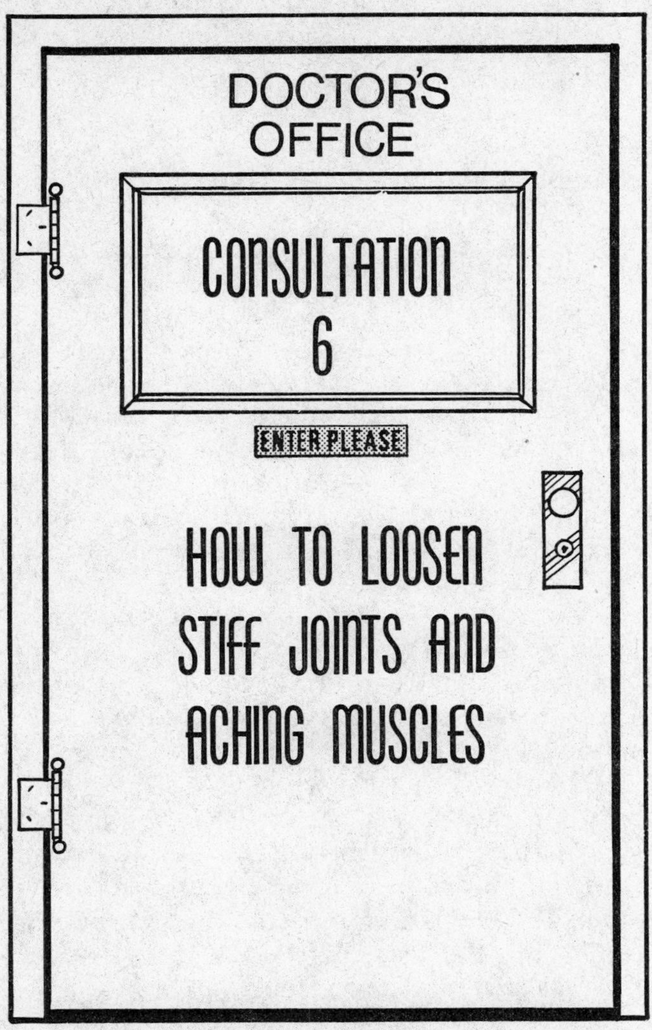

DOCTOR'S
OFFICE
CONSULTATION
6
ENTER PLEASE
HOW TO LOOSEN
STIFF JOINTS AND
ACHING MUSCLES

The Buddha Walk

The best approach to stiff joints and aching muscles is the gentle approach, the gradual approach. Do not engage in strenuous exercises in an attempt to correct either stiff joints or aching muscles. You may do serious damage to the joints and even produce an irreversible condition.

To accomplish the gentle, painless, safe approach to stiff joints and aching muscles, I have devised what I call the Buddha Walk. The Buddha, as a matter of interest to those of you who may not know, lived in India 600 years before Christ was born. He enunciated the golden rule 600 years before Christ. I tell you this to indicate that he was a man of great philosophical and spiritual stature and a man who developed a written philosophy that has passed down through the ages and is practiced to this day, not only in China and Japan but throughout the world. He walked, followed by his disciples, for many thousands of miles, and so the gentle philosophy of Buddha and the practice of walking, learning and teaching, has given me the name, "The Buddha Walk."

My version of the Buddha Walk is not designed for spiritual or religious purposes. It is designed entirely to reflect the spirit of a mind-body approach. You are now well aware that all my teachings, my practice of medicine and surgery, my books, have been devised with the sense that the mind and the body are one and must be treated as one. This can be called psychosomatic medicine, or holistic medicine.

To practice the Buddha Walk you walk slowly, with your hands clasped gently behind your back, the body erect, the shoulders thrown back and your head in a straight line with the line of your back. While you walk, you count slowly, one count to each step: one. . two. . .three. . .four. . .five. . .six. . .seven. You do this for seven steps, and while taking these seven steps, you gradually breathe slowly but deeply, beginning with the lower part of your lungs, going on next to the middle part of your lungs and concluding with filling the upper part of your lungs. This is accomplished by letting out your abdomen with the first step or two. This fills the lower part of your lungs. With the next step or two, you continue the deep breathing expanding your chest. This fills the middle part of your lungs. To fill the upper part of your lungs you must, as you are walking with your hands clasped behind your back, gradually raise the clasped hands as high as they will go behind your back and then throw your shoulders back while continuing to breathe. More air will then enter your lungs, filling the upper part of your lungs. You should do this to the count of seven slow steps.

You should continue walking for two steps while holding your breath and you will then for the next count of seven steps gradually let the air out of your lungs beginning above by lowering your clasped hands slowly, behind your back. You should then contract your chest muscles to empty the middle part of your lungs, and finally, you should contract your abdominal muscles to empty the air in the lower part of your chest.

This sounds and is very simple. However, until you have mastered it, you may find some difficulty in two ways. First, you may find difficulty in the measured step, in counting with each step, while filling the lungs from below upward. This will be a new way of breathing for most of you, and certainly a new way of combining a walking pace with breathing. Nevertheless, you must keep after it, since this is a most important exercise. Not only will it fill your lungs with energy and oxygen as you breathe deeply, but you will be filling parts of your lungs that you may scarcely have used at all, especially the upper part of your lungs. When you have completed the Buddha Walk to the point of the complete expiration of air, you again hold your breath for two steps before repeating the cycle of seven walking steps while drawing air into your lungs from below upward.

The Buddha Walk is to be continued for twenty to thirty minutes each day, preferably in the morning, immediately after breakfast. You may, of course, do this as often as you wish throughout the day, but one such walk per day is absolutely essential. I prefer the walk after breakfast as the essential one, and try to repeat the Buddha Walk throughout the day two or three additional times before bedtime.

The Buddha Walk is not designed for simply loosening stiff joints or aching muscles. It requires the full attention of the mind as well as the body, and the counting combined with the breathing empties the mind of otherwise potentially disturbing thoughts relating to the problems of that day, the problems of the past, and your anxieties about the future. When you become expert in the Buddha Walk, you will not only loosen stiff joints and aching muscles, but your emptied mind will now be able to give full attention to whatever you see around you. The colors of flowers, plants, trees, the texture and beauty of your surroundings, the blue sky, the clouds—whatever you may encounter during the walk—will now be appreciated with greater intensity than ever before.

You will use no words to describe what you see. The emptied mind, giving full attention to what you see, hear and smell, will experience much more fully if no words are used in description.

Since your mind will be occupied with the repetition of counting and the breathing itself, there will be no room for any other words. You will simply be seeing, feeling, hearing and sensing in every possible fashion with great intensity. The world will be much more beautiful for you during this time than it ordinarily is for the average person who is simply walking.

††*How Andrew J. Strengthened Lungs and Body*

I have taught the Buddha Walk to literally thousands of patients. Andrew J. illustrates the value of the Buddha Walk in terms of strengthening both lungs and body functions. Naturally, Andrew J., like all the other patients, was also taking the Revitalization Cocktail and following the Revitalization Plan at the same time. Therefore, we must attribute any and all improvement to the total plan as well as to the Buddha Walk.

Andrew J. practiced the Buddha Walk immediately after breakfast as instructed for a period of three months. He then found time to do the same thing after lunch and repeated it once again for thirty minutes before dinner. He felt that these were "the most important and helpful times of my life." He also told me, "Never have I more fully appreciated the beauty of trees and sky, never had I more fully appreciated everything I saw and heard and felt than I have during the times of the Buddha Walk." During these times he was fully relaxed, in a state of total passive awareness of everything about him, without any anxiety.

Before beginning this program, he was in the early stages of emphysema, with difficulty in getting enough air into his lungs, but not yet so far advanced that his lungs were useless. Naturally, he had been a heavy smoker all his life, and as part of the Revitalization Plan, he had given up smoking altogether. This helped enormously in conjunction with the Buddha Walk and deep breathing. His family physician and his internist found that his lungs improved greatly at the same time that his general health had improved.

He now had sufficient energy to walk great distances without shortness of breath, to enjoy his work and to enjoy his life at home. He had given up sex long before coming to see me, since it required "too much work." After one year of practice of the Buddha Walk, his body energy was sufficiently revitalized that he resumed sex with his wife with great pleasure and had become both in appearance and in function a very much younger man. This was quite an accomplishment for a man who began this practice at sixty years of age.

The Buddha Dance for Renewed Energy, Lung and Muscle Strength

The Buddha Dance is designed to do many things. It improves your capacity for relaxation, makes your muscles and joints more flexible, improves muscle capacity for lifting or other work, and renews energy. People who could not maintain ordinary calisthenic gymnasium-type exercises for more than a few minutes without exhaustion, can do the Buddha Dance for hours at a time and are completely relaxed, at ease and breathing easily at the end of that time. Even the heart muscle is strengthened, and a previously rapid heart rate can be ultimately reduced to a more normal pace. The Buddha Dance, therefore, is of great importance for all of you and is a major part of the Revitalization Program.

You may practice the Buddha Dance with music that you hear within yourself if you wish, or you can use a record player or FM radio station that plays good dance music. Indeed, one can dance to any type of music. If you wish, you may hum to yourself while dancing and provide your own musical accompaniment to the dance. You may practice the Buddha Dance in any room of your house, or outdoors if you are fortunate enough to have a sheltered terrace or some other area where you will not be concerned about onlookers.

The Buddha Dance is free-form dancing. Forget about fox trots, tangos and the like. You will not dance any of these types of dance steps. You will simply let your muscles relax and let yourself go in time with the music. As you dance, and you should begin the dancing relatively slowly if you have any physical problems with breathing, muscle strength or stiff joints, you gradually increase the pace of the dance and the use of various parts of the body, until all of your body is moving gracefully, smoothly, floating through the air.

If any of your muscles or joints are stiff, the increase in movement of these muscles and joints, as you dance about the room or elsewhere, must be very gradual. Do not press such muscles and joints to the point of severe pain. If you do it gradually, these stiff muscles will slowly relax, and you will sometimes be surprised at how rapidly this will occur. The same thing applies to joints that have been stiffened by disuse. Obviously, your breathing will not be very deep during this time, and you are not to practice the Buddha Walk type of breathing while dancing. Your breathing while doing the free-form dancing that I have called The Buddha Dance will be normal and not increased beyond the requirements of the dance itself.

Dancing in this fashion, once you have learned to do it with great ease, freedom of motion and spontaneity, empties the mind of troubled thoughts. You will find joy and beauty in the dance. When you have danced for a half-hour, later for an hour and sometimes longer, you will find yourself relaxed, not short of breath and with every muscle of your body limp and loose but fully under your control. Joints that were moving with difficulty before will now have a wider range of motion.

The Buddha Walk and the Buddha Dance are both of enormous importance in the Revitalization Program. Do not neglect these important mind-body exercises. Practice them both each day, as often as you can.

An excellent approach to free-form dancing for those who are not accustomed to dancing or who have stiff joints and/or aching muscles, is to simply walk around the room in time to the music. If the music is too fast for you, you may walk in half-time or as slowly as your condition demands. Do not push yourself until you limber up. Then, you may increase the pace of dancing little by little. You must avoid increasing the muscle or joint pain, if this is your problem. After you have become accustomed to the walking rhythm in time with the music, whether it be by slow steps or in time, you may then begin swaying your body from side to side as you walk. The next stage is when you add the movement of your arms and hands. You do this by imagining that you are the conductor of the orchestra. Now, your entire body is engaged in rhythmic, pleasurable motion. You are performing the Buddha Dance.

The final step, as you dance, is to repeat, in your mind, "younger, younger, younger, younger. . .healthier, healthier, healthier, healthier. . .happier, happier, happier and happier." As you dance, your entire body-mind becomes one with the music and with life itself. You will find this ultimate stage a time of true joy.

††*How a Doctor Learned to Relax and Enjoy Life*

One of my patients, a doctor who had required surgery for prolapse of the rectum (a condition that he had tolerated since 12 or 13 years of age until I operated upon him at age 45), was very tense, worked very hard in his practice (pediatrics) and had lost all capacity to enjoy his life. He had a fine wife and two children, but unfortunately, one of the children was retarded. This naturally soured his outlook on life, particularly since he was a pediatrician. We became good friends after I had operated on his prolapse and corrected it, and I told him of the Buddha Walk, the Buddha Dance and various meditation techniques that I had devised. I told him of the entire Revitalization Program. Gradually, he became interested and was soon following the entire program.

He learned to relax so that he could put his body in a total state of relaxation almost instantly. This could then be followed by either a nap for an hour or two, a deep sleep without dreams, or a full night's sleep—again, without dreams. He learned to put his mind so completely at rest by using the meditation formulas such as, "better and better, healthier and healthier, stronger and stronger, younger and younger," that he fell asleep as soon as he wished, almost always within five minutes after relaxing and beginning the meditation formula at bedtime.

Despite the irreversible problem of a retarded child, he learned to face and accept the reality of life within his own family just as he did within his practice. He became very active in the treatment and research of retardation in children, and told me that he was only now, for the first time, truly living in the present and not at all in the past. He still had his worries about the future but was nevertheless learning to relax and enjoy life in the present.

††*How Irma N. Discovered a New World*

Irma N. was forty-three years of age, depressed, unhappy in every possible way, had never married and felt that life was not worth living. She worked as a waitress and said, "All I could think about all day is how much my feet hurt." She had been treated by many doctors and came to me because of bleeding from the lower bowel. A careful and complete study had found nothing other than protruding hemorrhoids and constipation.

Irma had tried every form of laxative and cathartic in the treatment of her constipation without much help. Indeed, she rarely moved her bowels more than once every four days, and it was always a hard, painful movement, accompanied by active bright red bleeding. I advised removal of the hemorrhoids and did this for her without delay.

I told Irma that she ought to consider finding a new job. I had discovered, during our post-operative conversations, that she had other talents. She could type reasonably well, and I suggested that she might want to go back to a typing or secretarial school and learn how to use the more modern IBM typewriters. She was intelligent, and in my opinion, too intelligent to be working as a waitress. What she needed was a new approach to life, contact with people of better intellect than the average person she waited upon and with whom she actually had no real contact. She needed to talk to people with more interest in life that might be communicated to her simply by contact with them. Obviously, there is a great deal more to life than simply carrying food to a table and then carrying the empty plates back to the kitchen with new orders, repeating this throughout three meals a day. She had a better mind than that and needed to discover a new world.

I also advised her that she would do well to stop eating the type of food she was serving to her customers, since it was typical restaurant food full of fat, sugar, starches and, most likely, many harmful additives. She needed to lose weight, since she was eating almost constantly during the day, which had added unneeded pounds to her weight. I told her that if she practiced proper nutriton, her entire body would be more relaxed, her outlook on life would be more open and meaningful and she would have greater vitality. This change in appearance and energy would no doubt bring her into still further contact with the outside world and might possibly even find her a husband and a home.

She began to show interest in my ideas and gradually entered into the Revitalization Plan. She did indeed lose weight and showed signs of greatly increased energy as well as a new interest in the world. Her next step was to enroll in and attend a secretarial school, and she found the challenge and the companionship a still further discovery and pleasure. I wish that I could say she also found a husband and began a family life, but to my best knowledge that never did occur. However, she had in many ways truly discovered a new world both within herself and outside herself.

I do want to stress one point. Each person's world is chiefly within their own mind-body. Your world is totally unique and different from mine. If you want to discover a new world, you may need to change your occupation, make new contacts, attend schools or learn to enjoy books and the theatre. Whatever you have to do depends upon where you live and what your present interests are. There are many new worlds to discover and many ways to discover them. When you do this, you will internalize your discovery and will be living in a "new world."

The Half-Hour Flexercise

The half-hour flexercise is a technique that you can use at any time of the day, but one that you will find particularly helpful at any time that you are under stress, and certainly before going to sleep. The half-hour flexercise can be practiced while sitting in a chair, while standing or while lying down. To understand this type of exercise you must realize that you can literally "point your mind" to any muscle in your body, tell that muscle to contract or relax and it will do so. Try this with your hand muscles first, since this will most obviously prove my point. Tell your hand to form a fist and you will see that the muscles of your hand promptly respond. Now tell your hand muscles to relax and they will open and lie loose upon your lap or at the side of your leg if you are standing. You see, you do have control over your muscles. But regrettably, most of us let our muscles control us, and when we lose control, the result may be stiff joints and aching muscles. Furthermore, stiff joints and aching muscles produce a feeling of tension, anxiety and stress in all parts of the body-mind.

Now, let us try lying down flat on the back and practicing the flexercise procedure. Begin with your toes. Tell them to flex. They will flex back and forth as you tell them to. Now your feet. Ask your feet to move upward, bending toward the leg at the ankle and then downward—all the way downward until they are pointing straight ahead of you. Those muscles will do exactly as your mind directs.

Now, without moving the joints of your ankle or your knees, point your mind to the muscles in the back of your legs and tell them to contract and relax. You will be able to contract and relax these muscles at will, simply by this instruction from your mind. Keep practicing the contraction and relaxation of these muscles.

After a time, move on to pointing your mind at the muscles in front of your legs and put your hands on these muscles, so you can feel them tensing and relaxing as you tell them to do so. Do this without moving your feet, your ankles or your knees. Now do the same with the muscles in front of your thighs. Put your hands on them so that you can feel them contract and relax as you tell them to do so. They will do exactly as you command. Now, do this with the muscles at the side of your legs. They will do the same, and at the same time the buttock muscles will usually contract and relax. You can feel them do this with your hands.

Now, move your abdominal muscles. Do the same thing. Practice contracting and relaxing those muscles while your hands rest upon them and can feel this contraction and relaxation. In time, you will even learn how to roll those muscles by beginning the contraction low and gradually rolling the muscles upward to the base of the chest.

Now, let your hands lie at your sides, and do the same thing, beginning with your finger muscles. Contract and relax. Then bend your wrists and relax. Now, contract the muscles between the wrists and the elbows without moving the wrist and the elbow; just tell them to contract and relax and they will do so. Now, do the same with the muscles in front of your arm above the elbow. These muscles too will contract and relax as you point your mind at them. Repeat this with the muscles in back of your arm between the elbow and the shoulder.

Now, do this with your shoulder muscles and—if you wish—you may roll your shoulders in a circle backward and then forward, or just backward for a period of time, then forward for a period of time. This will contract and relax those muscles and simultaneously give you the flexercise type of movement of the shoulder joint itself.

Now, move to your forehead and contract your forehead to wrinkle it. Tell it to relax. The relaxed forehead is essential for total relaxation of the body and for sleep. Do the same thing with the circle of muscles around your eyes. Contract those until your eyes are tightly closed and then relax them. It is very important that these muscles be fully relaxed in order to have a quiet mind and a good night's sleep. Now, do the same with the muscles around your lips. There is a circle of muscles here that will purse your lips. And now relax those muscles. These muscles also must be fully relaxed in order to sleep peacefully, quietly, with total body-mind relaxation—often a dreamless sleep. You have now completed the half-hour flexercise. When you learn to do these things—the Buddha Walk, the Buddha Dance, the half-hour flexercise, you will realize that your mind and body are one. You will realize that your mind acts on the body and the body acts on the mind, since they are one. You will now fully understand why it is so important that both the mind and the body (the mind-body) must work in concert to relax if you are to release yourself from stress.

††*How Jacob R. Conquered Arthritis*

Arthritis is a complex disease that takes many forms. I urge you to write to The Arthritis Foundation, 475 Riverside Drive, New York, New York 10027, and ask for a booklet entitled, "Home Care Programs In Arthritis." Since each arthritis condition is unique and each individual patient is also unique, it is most important that your physician determine for you what type of arthritis you have and suggest the appropriate treatment. It is best, of course, if the physician who treats you is a specialist in this disease.

What I am about to tell you about Jacob R. is unusual in my experience. I know of no specific nutritional treatment that will "cure" arthritis. For that matter, there are no specific drugs that will "cure" arthritis, to my knowledge. However, if you practice the types of exercises I have just suggested, and if you enter upon the Revitalization Program as described, the total effect will be helpful to strengthen your body, provide new energy and give you more control over your muscles and joints.

That was the case with Jacob R., who suffered from a form of arthritis called "rheumatoid arthritis." I cautioned him that once he started on this program, he had to continue it forever. In addition, he had to be under the care of his arthritis specialist or internist. He agreed to follow these instructions. Although he had been taking medications for some time for his arthritis, he felt that he was becoming less and less capable of moving about without pain and more and more fearful that he would require major surgery to keep going. I explained to him that this was not my field, and that although there is no known "cure" for arthritis, he must keep himself as relaxed as possible, keep his hopes high and follow the appropriate instructions to reenergize his body and follow whatever treatment his doctor outlined for him.

What we did accomplish with the Revitalization Plan was a return of energy, a restoration of hope, a decrease of pain in the involved joints and improvement in motion and stability of those joints. During the six years that Jacob R. was under observation by his own physicians as well as myself, he seemed to show continuing improvement and was a much healthier, happier person than when I first saw him. He had, from his own point of view, "conquered arthritis."

I want to stress to you, as does The Arthritis Foundation and all physicians who practice the treatment of arthritis as a specialty, that it is possible to largely prevent the crippling and deforming effects of rheumatoid arthritis. You must be very patient in following any program that may be outlined by your physician, whether he is a specialist in arthritis or your family physician. You must be very patient and careful in following the Revitalization Program as I have outlined, since nutrition is important for the health of your muscles and joints as well as every other part of your body-mind. I strongly urge that with your practice of the Buddha Walk, the Buddha Dance and the half-hour flexercise, you also add, "Better and better, healthier and healthier, happier and happier," to your program of living, walking, eating and always before sleeping.

A final word of hope, a great deal can be done for arthritis, most of the crippling can be prevented, many of the problems now present can be corrected or improved upon, you can control the pain, and if you begin your treatment early enough, there will be no irreversable damage to joints.

††*Your Instructions For Today. . .*

1. **Practice the Buddha Walk each morning without fail.**
2. **Practice the Buddha Dance as often as you can each day, to strengthen muscles and loosen stiff joints.**
3. **The daily practice of both, combined with the Flexercise procedures, will teach you relaxation and muscle and joint control and will strengthen your mind-body approach to new health.**
4. **With total muscle-body-mind control, you will restore energy, confidence and capacity for joy in living.**

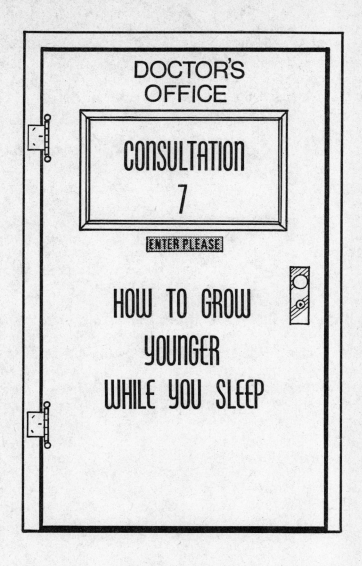

We have already discussed the repetition of words that will assist your body in reversing aging and in attaining new youth and greater vitality. The meditation formulas I will now discuss are comparable to those you have already learned in this book during our consultations. When you practice the art of meditation, you are practicing a form of positive thinking that is thousands of years old. It was practiced by our greatest religious leaders and by scientists throughout the centuries. Some went off into the "wilderness" or even lived in remote caves, to practice meditation throughout the entire day, every day, while others set aside special parts of the day to practice meditation. The modern methods now taught throughout the world by various schools of thought are all based upon these ancient techniques.

Meditation Formulas

There are two basic concepts that you should understand about meditation. One concept leads to the form of meditation that results in an *understanding* of the content of your mind. The mind, after all, as it involves the brain, is simply a most amazing, compact computer. This computer begins to receive information and store it from the moment we are born to the moment we die. Some of the information is useful throughout a lifetime, while other information becomes obsolete with the passage of time.

If we were to compare the brain as a computer with the various computers in use in business firms throughout the world, we would have to understand that the business type computer has its information changed as it becomes outdated. If the computer lists names and addresses, or methods of approach to particular problems, and the people whose names and addresses are listed have died or changed their location, and the methods of approach to problems have changed with new technology, this information is removed from the computer. The newer information is placed into the computer.

With the human mind it is a different matter. All the information, all the experiences that you have had throughout your entire lifetime, are permanently in your computer data banks. The only way you can obtain access to this information, most of which is stored at the unconscious level of the brain, is by understanding what that content is. Once you understand it, it will not be erased, but if it is outdated, you will no longer use it. It will no longer affect the way you think, the way you behave and the way you relate to the world. I have taught you ways to understand, insofar as that is possible, that there is certain information that does not help you in maintaining youth or restoring vigor and energy to prematurely aging tissues and organs of your body.

The second type of meditation is simply the use of phrases,

words, ideas that will add a positive type of programming to your mind at the conscious level as well as the unconscious level. When you use these phrases such as, "Better and better, healthier and healthier, younger and younger," regularly throughout your daily life activities, or at stipulated intervals such as in the morning upon awakening or in the evening before falling asleep, you will be consciously occupying your mind with reenergizing thoughts. Your mind cannot be in two places at once, and the use of this type of meditation formula involves both the mind and the body as a unit in the effort to revitalize and restore youth to your prematurely aging or ill body. Please follow the instructions I have already given you for the use of these formulas during our previous consultations.

We will, in the remainder of this consultation, give you examples of people who have benefitted greatly from these formulas, and show you how you can use them before sleep to overcome insomnia and to literally reverse the aging process. You can even use the formulas to program your body-mind toward the loss of excess weight while sleeping.

††*How Sylvia R. Discovered Reality and Happiness*

This patient came to me for various gastrointestinal complaints, and intensive examination by various consultants as well as by myself could show no organic basis for her problems. It was evident that she was living in a state of considerable stress, and it was also evident that she needed help in many ways.

Sylvia R. was in her early thirties, but had had a very unhappy childhood, a broken home and had never found it possible to relate to men. She therefore lived and worked alone, without pleasure and certainly without enjoyment of life. She took refuge in food and became extremely obese.

I explained to her that we could find nothing organic in our examinations, and that her basic problem was in the way she related to life. I also explained to her about the computer nature of her brain, and the fact that what she had experienced in her childhood and while growing up, the problems she had seen in the poor family relationship between her mother and father and such, had left her depressed with life itself and unhappy with other people, especially men. She could understand this and responded, "You would do the same thing if you had had the kind of life I had." No doubt she was right.

I told Sylvia that she was right, and that the answer was in understanding that the source of her problem went back into her childhood and throughout her life at home. She had unfortunately never had an opportunity to develop a more positive attitude toward life. I explained to her that she was living largely in the past, dwelling upon those days of great stress and serious problems, which colored all her actions to this very day. I continued to explain that once she understood this, as she apparently now did, she could begin to put happier, healthier, life-expanding thoughts into her computer brain, and in time, she would begin to put these new positive thoughts into action. When she did this she would see life differently, respond to people differently and begin to enjoy the present and anticipate a happier future.

I explained to her that the slow method of doing this would be through extensive psychoanalysis but that it would literally take years of talking about the past in the office of a psychiatrist. I told Sylvia that I had no objection to this technique if she wished to consult a psychiatrist. However, if she could simply understand, truly understand the concept of how her early programming was now acting to depress her view of life and if she could replace and reinforce her thoughts with appropriate new information that she would feed into her computer brain—this new, positive, living, hopeful, happy, life-restoring information would, in time, overshadow the depressing data programmed in her brain throughout her early life and up to this point.

She agreed that she would try. I then put Sylvia on the Revitalization Formula, told her of the entire Revitalization Plan, and advised her to practice repeating the following meditation formula while totally relaxed, before going to sleep at night and immediately upon awakening in the morning. She was also to repeat this meditation formula whenever she had a break during the day. Her formula was to be as follows, "I am becoming happier and happier, healthier and healthier, slimmer and slimmer, younger and younger, every day, in every way." I gave her detailed information on how to relax (just as you have learned in the previous six consultations).

Sylvia R. had truly understood. She put the meditation formulas and the Revitalization Program into action immediately. I had told her to come back in a month, but in two weeks she telephoned me to say that I had been right and that she was beginning to feel like a new person already. She couldn't wait to tell me that she had already become somewhat slimmer, although she had no scale to measure the weight loss.

I was delighted to hear this, and in succeeding consultations during the next six months, I learned that she was practicing the meditation formula each morning, during the afternoon "coffee break" at work and at night before going to sleep. She had become a totally different person in many ways. She had lost thirty pounds and was beginning to discover the world in a new way—finding a new reality—with happiness and the expectation of more happiness in the future.

Sylvia R. moved to the Midwest after the first year of our relationship and found a new world—a world that had opened up to her as soon as she had given up the depression and the problems of the past and had learned to live for the present moment. She had truly discovered a new reality and a new happiness. I do not know whether she ever married.

No-Dream Sleep

To sleep without dreams is to sleep without nightmares. Very few dreams are happy or constructive. Most, if remembered, are tormented and sometimes very frightening nightmares. If it were possible to sleep without dreams, the sleep would be at a deeper level, as has been proven by electroencephalograph studies made on patients during sleep. When a person is dreaming, the depth of sleep is much more shallow than when they are sleeping a dreamless sleep. It is that sleep which is most relaxed, in which the person moves about the least and from which he awakens the most refreshed. So, it is important to have sleep without dreams. But it is difficult for the average person. Once again, the relaxation methods and the meditation formulas, combined with the Revitalization Plan, offer the possibility for dreamless sleep to many patients.

I urge you to practice these techniques at every possible opportunity, even if it is only just before going to sleep at bedtime. Relax all your muscles, let yourself go limp and loose, and then tell yourself, "Happier and happier, healthier and healthier, younger and younger, every day in every way." Repeat this over and over again until you fall asleep. The very expectation of dreamless sleep, combined with the total relaxation of the body-mind and the positive program introduced by your meditation formula, will hopefully give you dreamless sleep through most of the night.

If you achieve this on a regular basis, much of the stress that is causing breakdown in your various tissues and organs, much of the anxiety that leaves you feeling pessimistic during the next day, will no longer exist. You will indeed be more relaxed, happier and healthier throughout the following day and every day.

††*How Martha L. Overcame Insomnia and Gained New Vitality*

Insomnia is a very common condition. When we are under stress, bedeviled by everyday anxieties and sometimes even by problems of the distant past or fear of the future, we often stay up at night, talking to ourselves, trying to solve problems that have not yet occurred or that are long past. Insomnia reduces our vitality, can cause premature aging and can even increase the possibility of a heart attack during sleep. It is a dangerous condition.

Many people with insomnia have attempted to help themselves by watching television for half the night, which merely increases the insomnia. They have then conditioned themselves to staying up later and later for the late show, then the late-late show, even to the point of watching an early morning show to keep them up until breakfast. I advise patients who do stay up to watch television until the late hours of the night that they are simply stimulating themselves and that this is precisely the opposite of what they should do if they wish to fall asleep. So, no late television shows if you have difficulty falling asleep. Instead of that, put yourself on the Revitalization Plan, add to it the meditation formulas for falling asleep and the important practice of the half-hour flexercise before falling asleep.

The half-hour flexercise is described, as you recall, in our sixth consultation. It gives you an objective in terms of an exercise that occupies both mind and body and results in ultimate relaxation. When you have completed the flexercise, begin talking once again to your mind-body, but this time start with the head. Tell your scalp to relax. Forehead to relax. Eyes relax. Cheeks relax. Mouth relax. These are the most important areas, and when you have relaxed the muscles around your eyes, your forehead and the muscles that purse your lips, you will be halfway toward deep relaxation and sleep.

Now continue—neck relax. Shoulders relax. Arms relax. Forearms relax. Hands relax. Pause at this time and say, "Deeper and deeper, deeper and deeper, deeper and deeper."

Now continue, chest relax, abdomen relax, buttocks relax, legs relax, feet relax—at that point you will find your entire body in a total state of relaxation.

You then repeat, "Deeper and deeper, deeper and deeper, every muscle in deeper and deeper relaxation."

Martha L. was a good student, intelligent and capable of following instructions. Within two weeks, she had kicked the television habit and found it possible to remain in a deep state of relaxation after beginning the relaxation exercise at ten o'clock in the evening. Her deep state of relaxation finally put her to sleep, as nearly as she can determine, toward midnight. At first, she slept only three or four hours, but after a time she had a full night's rest of six to eight hours' sleep.

††*How Lewis S. Learned to Roll with the Punches*

Lewis S. managed a supermarket. At first he objected when I told him about the requirements of the revitalization formula and the Revitalization Program. Lewis objected most strenuously when I told him that the supermarket products were to be avoided because they possibly contained injurious additives, often had large amounts of sugar in breakfast cereals and were certainly inadequate from the point of view of nutrition. The fact that when bread was stripped of its wheat germ and additives were put in to partially replace the loss did not make the bread a good product for adequate nutrition. The same applied to the breakfast cereals. Vitamins should not be additives to breakfast cereals.

I pointed out the importance of the larger levels of vitamins in accordance with the concept of an optimal level rather than a minimal or "required" level that simply maintain the body for a longer time before it falls apart. Lewis was an intelligent man and could understand. Indeed, since his job was to manage a supermarket and sell these very products to his customers, he had to learn to "roll with the punches" both during our discussions and when he first began the Revitalization Program.

In terms of his work, he realized that it was impossible to reconstruct the entire world and that the average person would still continue to buy in his supermarket. That did not mean that he had to be the average person. I had explained to him that we are each unique and that our requirements are unique. Lewis understood this, and followed through with the program with no difficulty at all. His problems were many—an overactive colon, a tendency to vomit after breakfast and before going to business and difficulty with sleep. He would wake frequently during the night, with desperate dreams about a lost job and failing health.

Careful examination revealed nothing more than an anxiety state, and I told him that his symptoms were stress-produced. He accepted this diagnosis, and after four months on the Revitalization Program, he had become adapted to his work and was sleeping better, with fewer dreams. Finally, one year later, with practically no dreams, he had regained much of the vitality that he had in his youth. In his early fifties, he now looked no more than forty, had a new bounce in his step and was bright and clear throughout the day, having slept well the night before.

The Isometric Pre-Sleep Procedure

Isometric exercises are useful before attempting sleep, but the type of exercise that I call "isometric" involves no movement of the joints. It is simply a matter of going into a state of deep relaxation and then "pointing the mind" to the muscles of the body, one at a time, and telling them to contract. I have already described this in Consultation 6. As a pre-sleep procedure, it helps to produce deep relaxation and provides healthy circulation by a form of exercise that is not fatiguing. This combination is exceedingly important, not only for deep relaxation, but for improved circulation and the ultimate slowing of the heart when the isometric exercises and the relaxation deepen immediately prior to falling into a deep sleep.

The sleep that results from the combination of this procedure and one of the meditation formulas such as, "Healthier and healthier, younger and younger, healthier and healthier, younger and younger. . ."will produce not only deep relaxation of the body, but also produces relaxation of the mind. The mind, occupied with the repetition of this meditation formula, cannot, at the same time, concern itself with anxieties of the past, of the present or of the future. This isometric pre-sleep procedure has been most helpful to me personally, and I can vouch for its effective result in terms of deep and usually dreamless sleep.

††*How Jack D. Found New Health and New Youth While Sleeping*

This rapidly aging patient, Jack D., was in his early fifties and looked as if he were in his late sixties. He was engaged in the real estate business and was very successful and wealthy. It would seem, from my vantage point, that he had nothing to worry about finally. However, he told me that all was not as it seemed on the surface, and he was always heavily in debt to banks and others. In any case, he was living well, but perhaps beyond his means. Certainly, based on what he told me, his wife and two daughters were living beyond his means. To make matters worse, he had a mistress, and it appeared that her demands were also extreme. I suggested that he would need to change his lifestyle.

I advised Jack to decide between the stress produced by a mistress and the advantages that might overbalance that stress. In my opinion, the stress was aging him prematurely, and I could not imagine that the mistress had enough to offer to warrant this type of self-destruction. As for his wife and daughters and their spending habits, I suggested that he speak with them and tell them what the facts of life were. I was certain that if they loved him or had any concern for him at all as a person, they would cooperate and learn to live within their means. Finally, because he was compensating for all his problems by excessive eating of very high-fat French foods, I strongly urged that he place himself immediately on the Revitalization Plan.

Jack also suffered from insomnia, as he well might with all these problems. On the basis of this knowledge I suggested that he sleep in a separate bedroom, and when I made this suggestion I found that he had been sleeping in a separate bedroom for the past two years, simply because his wife liked to watch television until late at night. I then told him that this would help provide the opportunity to fall asleep much earlier than usual, and described to him the various techniques for attaining a dream-free sleep. His meditation formula was to be, "Younger and younger, slimmer and slimmer, healthier and healthier."

This was a remarkable patient who knew how to follow instructions and was dependable in every way. He did exactly as I ordered, placed himself on the proper diet, went to bed at an early hour each evening, and was soon sleeping very well indeed, at least eight hours a night. Jack came to see me one month later, saying that the program was a "revelation" to him and that he no longer suffered from insomnia. He did miss the French food, since the Revitalization Plan did not offer this type of "luxury" and self-destruction. However, he realized that it was a form of suicide, and gradually lost his taste for high-fat food. It took a full year before he had begun to show the signs of renewed health and renewed youth. The ultimate result was a happier and healthier man, much younger in appearance and definitely much younger in terms of his cardiovascular system.

††*Your Prescription for Today...*

1. **Practice the meditation formulas as often as you can, at least in the morning after waking.**
2. **If you have difficulty falling asleep or have disturbing dreams, practice the meditation formula before sleep and combine it with the isometric pre-sleep procedure.**
3. **If you wish to grow younger while you sleep, lose weight while you sleep and revitalize your body while you sleep, the combination of the various suggestions given to you during this consultation make up your prescription for today.**

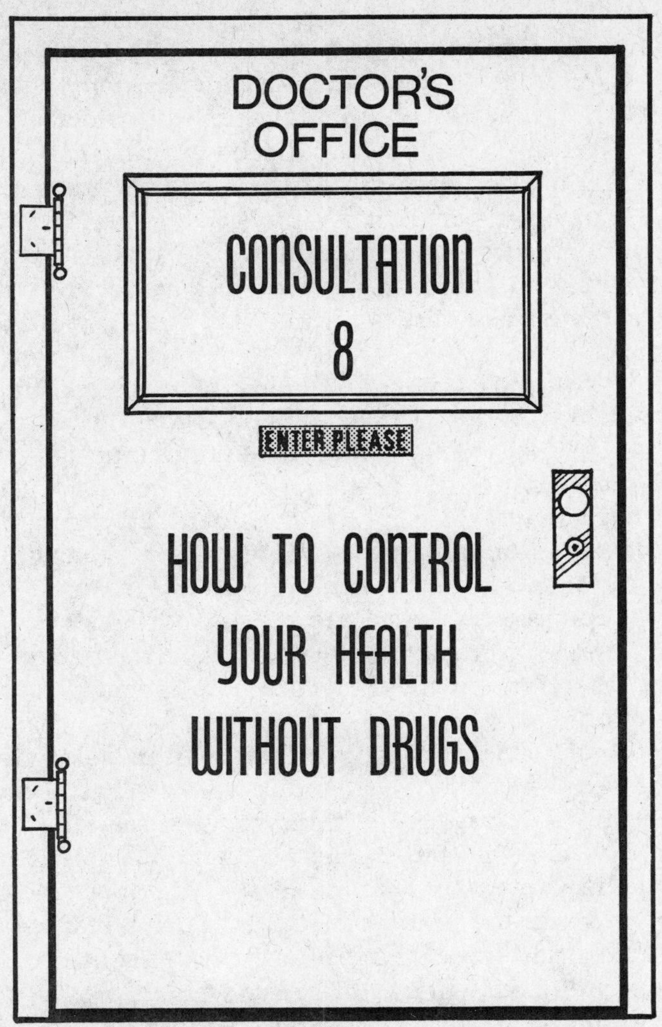

Drugs Versus Diet

Proper nutrition, combined with exercise and a positive attitude toward life, will do more to restore good health, maintain good health, prolong life and even revitalize an already damaged body than drugs will. By drugs, I refer to chemical compounds sold either over-the-counter or by prescription. Naturally, I believe that the patient should always have an accurate diagnosis when he feels ill or when there is some obvious disturbance that calls for either medical or surgical care. Once the diagnosis is made, the patient should follow the advice of his physician. To aid the physician in achieving better health or restoration to a normal state, it is my opinion that the body cells, tissues and organs must be provided with the best possible nutrients so that they may adequately respond to the physician's care.

In my own practice, there have been thousands of patients with constipation as a major symptom. And yet, I have never prescribed laxatives or cathartics. Proper diet will do more to establish a normal bowel habit than drugs. In all cases, I hasten to add, the correct diagnosis must first be made, since constipation can be a problem of serious dimensions, perhaps the result of a possibly malignant obstruction. But, once the diagnosis is made and there is no evidence of organic disease, I prefer to use the Revitalization Plan nutrition in the treatment of constipation, rather than laxatives or cathartics. During our first consultation, you learned of patients who had hardening of the arteries, obesity and physical depression. All were treated with drugs of one type or another before starting on the Revitalization Program. The drugs were not effective; the Revitalization Program, without drugs, was effective.

In the second consultation, you will recall a patient with angina pectoris resulting from spasm and partial closure of the arteries of the heart, a patient with intermittent claudication or spasms of the arteries of the legs and patients with high blood pressure, on the verge of stroke, all of whom had been under medical care with prescribed medications. The drug treatment did help to control pain to some degree and there was some lowering of blood pressure in patients with elevated blood pressure, but treatment without drugs or in conjunction with optimal nutrition for the mind and body, seemed to be even more effective. Throughout all the consultations in this book, I describe patients with exactly the same response when dealing with control of their health without drugs. Again, I must caution you. This is not to say that *all* disease will respond to treatment without drugs; even surgery may be necessary. There are many drugs produced by ethical pharmaceutical manufacturers and prescribed by physicians that are very helpful, often essential and indeed life-saving in many cases. You must always see your physician first, avoid self-treatment and follow his instructions.

Emptying Bowel, Bladder and Brain of Self-Destructive End-Products

It is impossible to be entirely well unless you have developed the habit of emptying your bowel, bladder and brain regularly each day. We will go into this in greater detail, but the principle is simple, and should be obvious to you.

The function of the bowel and the bladder is to empty the body of waste products. These waste products, if retained in the body, are toxic. Toxic products, whether coming from the outside through pollution of the air you breathe or from adulteration of the food you eat, poison and age the body. They reduce energy and decrease your capacity for long life. Toxic products are formed in the body as well as taken in through the respiratory tract and through the mouth. The French saying, "Death enters through the mouth," is very true. It also enters through the respiratory tract, through the nose, through the skin (excessive exposure to sunlight) and especially through the foods we eat. For revitalization (rejuvenation) of body tissues, you must avoid all toxic products in the air and in your food and water, and you must simultaneously empty your bowel and bladder of the toxic end products of digestion and other body functions on a regular basis.

We have spoken at length about this in Consultation 3, and you have learned the magic secret of bran, and the relationship of an empty bowel (regularly emptied each day) to the prevention and control of bowel infection, diverticulosis and diverticulitis, as well as the very common hemorrhoids (piles).

††*More About Bran—The Story of Pauline O.*

Ms. Pauline O. reversed aging and began to show tissue revitalization throughout her body when she added two heaping tablespoonfuls of wheat germ bran to her diet each morning. She used this bran as part of her Revitalization Cocktail, a cocktail consisting of one glass of orange juice, two heaping tablespoonfuls of bran, two heaping tablespoonfuls of sunflower seeds, and one level tablespoonful of wheat germ. At a later stage, I urged the addition of one heaping tablespoonful of lecithin granules. This mixture was placed in an Osterizer (there are many other brands of mixing devices that are equally suitable), and when thoroughly converted to liquid, it made a nutritious, revitalizing drink.

Pauline noticed that her skin assumed a healthy, bright tone. It was not the color resulting from exposure to the sun. Indeed, I advise all my patients to avoid more than twenty to thirty minutes exposure to the sun each day, especially if they live in a tropical climate. Sunlight ages the skin. Pauline's skin really glowed with good health, wrinkles disappeared and her forehead and the area around her eyes became smooth. Her eyes appeared more brilliant, and she thought that even her vision had improved. Her evaluation of her own state of health, after being on this simple regime for six months, was that she had become "twenty years younger." Indeed, she looked it, and her previously elevated blood pressure had also returned to a more normal average level.

The bran resulted in an easy emptying of the bowel each morning, and "pile protrusions" became a thing of the past. She was no longer straining at stool. The total result could be called revitalization of bowel function, skin health, arterial wall health (lowering the blood pressure) and a general tonic effect upon the entire body and mind. One year later, at age 66, I suggested that Pauline add five grams of vitamin C to her Revitalization Cocktail. Using 500 mg. tablets, this meant ten tablets added to her cocktail. In effect, I was advocating fortified orange juice for its vitamin C actions. You may, of course, use grapefruit or any other fruit juice, if you prefer.

During the cancer danger age, which probably begins quite early in life, it is best to take preventive measures. One of these preventive measures is—in my opinion—a large dose of vitamin C each day. Vitamin C is a natural food, and I personally take ten grams each day, five grams with my morning Revitalization Cocktail and five grams in orange juice as my second Revitalization Cocktail about mid or late afternoon. You might consider doing the same. To refresh your memory on vitamin C and other vitamins, I would suggest that you turn back to your fourth consultation and read about vitamins for prevention and disease control as well as the important effects of vitamins in mega dosage.

How to Empty Your Brain and Be Born Anew Each Day

It is exceedingly important to have an empty brain as well as an empty bowel and an empty bladder. How can this be accomplished. I have written three books on this subject, and it is obviously very difficult to compress the information of three books into a few paragraphs.

However, as a starter, let us consider the fact that the brain is very much like a computer. It is filled with data from infancy on. Most of that data is fed into the brain-computer by authority figures such as mother, father, older brothers and sisters, teachers, etc. Some of it is very useful information, and helps us in survival as well as in our revitalization project. However, much of the information becomes rapidly outdated, and some of it instills fears, anxieties and stress factors that actually wear us down at an emotional level throughout a lifetime. Anything that affects the emotions affects all other parts of the body. When you are afraid, for example, certain hormones are released through the body, blood pressure goes up, the heart rate increases, adrenaline is secreted into the blood stream and we are ready for either "fight or flight." This was a survival reaction when we lived in the jungle. It is not a survival reaction when we live in so-called "civilization," although much of our civilization remains a jungle, particularly the large urban centers of the world.

Certainly we cannot live without stress. A small amount of stress is useful, but only if the reaction is not one of overreaction. When we react excessively, the result is destructive. When we react in moderation in response to a genuine threat, the result is constructive. Now, think of the fact that much of the data that has been fed into your computer-brain is now outdated. It may even be totally self-destructive. You may have been programmed to eat the wrong foods, perhaps to eat too much. Most mothers think that their children do not eat enough and literally stuff them with the wrong foods. Candy, cookies, cakes are rewards for being "good." Overstuffed children are thought to be healthy by their misguided parents. As a matter of fact, they are suffering from true malnutrition. My own mother gave me a chocolate laxative before I went to sleep each night. She then programmed me quite correctly by saying, "sleep in good health and wake up in good health." I did indeed sleep well, but the laxative had adverse effects over the years.

Now we come to the important question of how to empty your mind of such ideas, such self-destructive habits and concepts. The answer is that once you *understand* the content of the mind, you can readily cope with such ideas as you face them. You can recognize them for what they are—self-destructive garbage of the past. In computer language, "garbage in, garbage out." This means that if you feed erroneous data into a computer, only erroneous answers can come out. If you feed the garbage of "hate thy neighbor," "envy thy neighbor," greed, jealousy, bigotry, overeating or overmedicating into your data bank, only destructive behavior can result.

Now, if you recognize that this is what your mind contains, you will be ready to reject any such ideas and the actions suggested by such ideas that develop during the course of each day. Each time you *pause and think before acting,* evaluate your thoughts and the action suggested by those thoughts, you improve the content of your brain. The pause, the reflection and the evaluation, give you a chance to act constructively rather than simply react like a mechanical computer. The answer and the accompanying action that results will be less stressful, more constructive and less harmful to you and those about you.

How to Empty Your Brain Before Sleep

Before you fall asleep, review the events of the day. Review the important thoughts and actions of that day. Are you satisfied that you have acted in a civilized fashion in accordance with the precept, "love thy neighbor as thyself"? If not, try to understand why not. Try to see the relationship between your behavior and your teachings of the past. Once you understand this, you will have emptied your mind of such behavior and its consequences, and when you have reviewed the day thoroughly from beginning to end, you will be at peace with yourself. You will have emptied your brain for that day.

Make this a habit each night. If you have an opportunity to do so during the course of the day, you can do this at those times as well, but it is most important at night. A brain that is emptied at night before sleeping is a brain that permits you to sleep without anxiety and without sleeping pills or other drugs. It will be the most restful sleep you have ever had, and it is likely that you will not dream. If you do dream, the dreams will probably be pleasant. In any case, when you wake in the morning, your mind—emptied of the problems of the past—will be born anew. This is the best way to be born anew, and you can be born anew each day.

What is The Brain?

The emptied brain is most important. Let me tell you my concept of what the brain really is. It is not simply the content of the upper part of your skull. Of course, that is where most of brain does indeed lie as it relates to the recording of the past, the evaluation of the present and the future and planning for the future. However, in my opinion every cell of your body is part of the brain. If you lose a single finger, your "brain" is changed to that degree, and you are a different person. If you lose an arm or leg, again you have lost a large fraction of your "brain," and you will become a still more different person. If you lose the sight of one eye or both, or lose your hearing, each cell of those organs is a loss of part of your brain, and you have indeed become a different person. The content of your brain, in my concept of the brain, obviously determines what you are and how you behave.

As a matter of fact, each cell is an individual living unit that acts and reacts to determine its own vitality and the vitality of the tissues around it as well as those at a distance. The hormones of the body are secreted by the endocrine glands, such as the pituitary gland at the base of the brain (master gland), the thyroid gland at the base of the neck and the adrenal glands on the top of each kidney, which are all exceedingly important organs, each of which determines whether or not we function as a normal or average person, as a devitalized individual, or as a revitalized and rejuvenated person whose life span has been lengthened and whose quality of life has improved. Just think of the change that would take place in you if your thyroid gland ceased to function. The absence of these few cells at the base of your neck would change you into a cretin, a veritable vegetable. The brain in the upper part of your skull would no longer function adequately, and you would function on a moronic level or not at all.

So, you see, I consider every cell of your body a part of the brain, and you must revitalize each cell, each organ, each tissue, every single part of your body if you wish to become happier, healthier, younger.

Revitalization Without Drugs

The revitalization begins by removing the destructive or self-destructive thoughts and programmed habits in your brain, replacing them with an understanding of the content of your brain and how it got to be the way it is. Then, after emptying the self-destructive data, replace that data with constructive, positive action toward a life based upon "love thy neighbor" instead of "beggar thy neighbor" and with revitalizing habits of eating and living. You may be surprised to find that when you try to understand another person, when you show concern for their well being or compassion for their needs, you will be repaid in kind and will become a happier, healthier, revitalized individual.

Remember, if you want to control your health and revitalize your body, you must learn to empty the bowel, empty the bladder and empty the brain daily.

††*How One Patient Stopped Smoking and Started Living*

Now, since most of the patients I speak with have a smoking habit, I do want to give you a few more words of caution. Let me do it in terms of a case history. Jerry T. smoked two packs a day. Judging from his behavior in my office, I think he probably smoked even more. He was nervous, constantly jerking about while sitting in my consulting room, and his obvious inability to control smoking (no smoking is permitted in my office), was not only making him a nervous wreck, but wasn't doing me any good as well. I told him that he could not possibly be revitalized while he was poisoning himself with nicotine. The smoke itself, plus the nicotine and whatever else it is in tobacco that causes cancer of the lung and hypertension in terms of high blood pressure and stress, act together to devitalize the body. He had come to me because he heard that I had a method to revitalize (he used the word "rejuvenate") any person, no matter how "far gone" they were. Naturally, I do not have any such method for those who are "too far gone." However, regardless of your condition, you can certainly be helped to some degree.

I advised Jerry that until he stopped smoking, very little of what I had to offer would be helpful to him. He was forty years old at the time, a top executive in a multi-million dollar business, and believed his work was both a social and a physical necessity. I pointed out the dangers of smoking not only in terms of his present condition, but in terms of the ever-present danger of cancer of the lung. I told him that cancer of the lung was the major cancer in the male patient, and that if he developed such a cancer he had only a 7 percent chance of living five years after surgery (assuming that he survived the very extensive surgery required). If the cancer had already spread to other parts of the body, he would probably die within the first six months after surgery. I asked him to consider his body as a corporation consisting of many cells trying to work together to produce a successful business—a happy, healthy, revitalized corporation. He could see this, he could understand this. I then told him that destructive thinking, bad habits and self-destructive data from the past which were fed into his receptive brain at a time when the computer brain was unable to evaluate for itself, were the cause of his present smoking. Indeed, now that he knew the correct data, and since he was otherwise extremely intelligent and constructive in his work, he should know that if he continued smoking, he would only be working toward the destruction of the corporate structure known as his body. This, too, was language that he understood. I told him that, in my opinion, the only way to stop was to stop all at once and "lick the habit by understanding it." This, I felt, was particularly true for a man of his intelligence. He could easily equate the important cooperative effort of every cell of his body to stay alive, to survive, to become stronger and healthier, with the type of effort he was putting into his corporate business. It was an appeal to his intellect, to his understanding, to his capacity as a top-level executive.

I told Jerry that I could do nothing more for him until he had "kicked the habit." When his body was again functioning cooperatively to survive rather than to self-destruct, I would be glad to take him on as a patient and show him the royal road to revitalization.

I did not see him again until six months later. At that time, he was completely self-controlled and a totally new person in every way. He had succeeded in understanding and acting upon his understanding. In his own way, he had been born anew that day and each day thereafter. I then put him on the revitalization program, and the results were remarkable in every way. His energy was enormous, his blood pressure returned to normal. His capacity for work became even greater than it was before, and he told me that his judgment was far superior to what it had been when he first visited my office. Jerry looked and acted as if he were a young man in his twenties.

Kicking the Additive Diet

I put all my patients on a diet that avoids additives insofar as additives can be avoided in this insane world. Our remarkable government—certainly one of the best in the world in its efforts to keep its citizens healthy, allows the smoking of cigarettes and merely adds a warning to the cigarette package that "tobacco may be injurious to your health," or words to that effect. Since tobacco not only may be injurious to your health, but is always damaging, and since it is the major cause of cancer of the lung, a totally deadly disease in both male and female (but especially in the male patient) and since nicotine and the other destructive products in cigarettes gradually destroy all the cells in the body in terms of their capacity for totally vitalized functioning, it seems curious that our government permits tobacco to be sold in any form.

But what about the additives in our foods? Once again, the government regulations strike a note that falls jarringly on the sensitive ear. Suspected cancer-causing chemicals are added to many products you find in the supermarket, from bacon to frankfurters to breakfast foods—ad infinitum. Even if you were to try to grow your own fruits and vegetables, you might find residual toxic products in the soil from atomic bomb explosions. The manufacturers who are interested in a long shelf-life for their products will put additives in their foods and remove those parts of the food that might shorten shelf-life. The portions removed are the best, most healthful parts of the foods. The additives are often cancer-causing.

The best I can offer you in terms of kicking the additive habit is to avoid starch and sugar in your diet. Do not eat prepared foods. Eat a natural, high-fiber diet. I personally obtain fiber from two or more tablespoonfuls of wheat germ bran each day (very inexpensive in a health food store) and several ounces of sunflower seeds that I mix with cottage cheese each day. My breakfast, as a matter of fact, consists of the Revitalization Cocktail—containing two heaping tablespoonfuls of wheat germ bran, one level tablespoonful of yeast flakes, one heaping tablespoonful of lecithin granules, five grams of vitamin C, one ounce of safflower oil and one large glass of orange juice (all well mixed in an Osterizer). I often add four tablets containing calcium and vitamin D to this. I obtain additional bran, together with many vitamins, in the sunflower seeds which I add to four or five large tablespoonsfuls of low-fat cottage cheese. I like the crunchy effect of chewing the sunflower seeds together with the cottage cheese. After this, I eat the whites of two hard-boiled eggs. That is my total breakfast.

Now, if I avoid starch foods and sugar-filled foods, I will largely avoid additives. If I obtain my protein from low-fat cottage cheese and the whites of hard-boiled eggs, I will again largely avoid additives. If I avoid prepared foods, I will avoid most food additives. If I am on a high-fiber diet, I will empty my bowel more rapidly each day, thus removing any additives that might have somehow gotten past the intellect and the mouth, so that they will have less opportunity to do damage within the intestinal tract of the body. That is about as far as we can go in terms of protecting ourselves against any money-oriented government that permits food producers to poison its citizens.

How Adrienn R. Lost Pounds and Freed Herself from Physical and Emotional Pressures

Adrienn was only 32 years old, but looked 50 and weighed as much as a professional wrestler. This was enough to disturb her both physically and emotionally. My problem was how to persuade Adrienn to eat properly, to think properly and to empty her brain of the self-destructive ideas that were presently destroying her health.

When a patient comes to me with these types of problems, they are obviously well motivated. That is the major key to whatever success I might have. It would do no good if I went out and sought people who were attempting suicide by overeating, eating the wrong foods, breathing noxious air, thinking self-destructive and society-destructive thoughts. But, those who are doing exactly these things and do come to me for help are the "suicidal" patients who want to be told how to avoid killing themselves. The fact that you are reading this book puts you in the well-motivated class and enormously increases your chance for a good result in revitalizing your body, restoring your health insofar as that is possible and adding years to your life.

I pointed out to Adrienn that she, and practically all my other patients, were attempting suicide. This was their way of killing themselves. She recognized and accepted this and asked me if I could tell her why she was attempting to commit suicide. Obviously, I could give her many routine stock answers. However, I told her simply that the answer was within herself, and that she must learn to understand how her mind works, what the content of her mind was. She would then know the answer, get rid of the causes of her emotional problems and immediately take the road to better health.

I told her about the content of the mind, not just her mind but every mind, including my own. I told her how the habits, the thoughts, the training that she received from infancy on, perhaps the overstuffing with food by an overprotective mother or father, might possibly have been factors in her present obesity problem. I told her that she must understand that the content of her mind was largely destructive, self-destructive, and she must go back into the past and consider what there was during that time, from infancy on, that might have started her on the road to self-destruction.

I told her to simply lie down in bed each night, about one-half hour before she expected to go to sleep, relax every muscle in her body and then let her mind go back to the past and remember the attitudes of her mother and father, other authority figures in the past, what types of foods they ate, the quantities, whether or not they urged her to eat fattening foods, starchy foods, high-sugar foods and so on. I then told Adrienn that she must empty her mind of all such instructions of the past. This was the "garbage in" of the computer phrase, "garbage in, garbage out." The "garbage out" was her obesity.

She understood this, and put this practice into effect. Naturally, at the same time I told her of the importance of the high-fiber, low-starch, low-sugar, no-prepared-foods diet. She understood this as well and proceeded accordingly. It was quite remarkable how her weight melted away without drugs and without counting calories. Indeed, she followed my own practice of breakfast and lunch or breakfast and dinner—two meals a day only. She enjoyed this. She had risen to the challenge, and had responded beautifully. Within seven months Adrienn had lost one-third of her previous weight and was not only slim but remarkably attractive, no longer tired and no longer disturbed by the emotional pressures of the past. And, she had learned to live one day at a time.

I had explained to her that until we forget the problems of the past and the fears of the future, and until we live only in the present, we are not truly living at all. She understood this and was, to the best of her ability, living in the present only. One year later, Adrienn was married. She then had a child of her own, and I do not doubt that she has been feeding that child a proper diet, as free from starch, sugar and additives as possible. She had revitalized her own body and no doubt had added years to her life.

††*A Simple Secret of Longevity—The Story of Harry K.*

This is the story of another top executive, Harry K., who improved both his business and his health by learning a simple secret of longevity. The body is made up chiefly of water, and this man drank practically no water. When he did, it was tap water. I told him about the toxic products in tap water, even at its best, and advised him to drink bottled hard water with a high mineral content. I gave him the name of a bottled spring water that I drink myself and buy for my family. He bought it by the gallon and drank it by the gallon, since I advised him to drink as much as one gallon a day.

Harry was not particularly ill when he came to see me, but he did feel that he lacked sufficient energy and wanted to prolong life if possible. I explained the importance of exercise and recommended the Buddha Walk described in Consultation 6. He loved that prescription, and was soon walking long distances. Fortunately, Harry lived well out on Long Island, away from the poisonous gases in the atmosphere of New York City. The Buddha Walk quieted his mind and strengthened his body. At the same time, it programmed his mind with the concept of better and better health and youth.

I advised him, since he found it necessary to have business luncheons each day, to eat half-portions, and to order in accordance with the dictum of "no starch or sugar and no prepared foods," he also understood and acted upon my suggestion for a high-fiber diet. The Revitalization Cocktail was a revelation for

Harry, and he enjoyed it each morning, following my breakfast pattern regularly. In addition, he took 800 I.U. of vitamin E and five grams of vitamin C each day. The vitamin E was taken by mouth directly in capsule form and the vitamin C was taken in his Revitalization Cocktail.

He boasted of his renewed energy, his greater capacity for work and, most of all, of the fact that he was enjoying life. Harry K. paid me a great compliment when he said that I had "given him a new lease on life."

††*How One Patient Avoided a Second Coronary and Restored His Youth*

Most physicians see patients who come near to death after suffering a coronary occlusion (clot closure of one of the arteries that brings blood to the heart muscle). However, most physicians also see these patients die of a second coronary not too long after the first. Sid J. avoided a second coronary, and indeed became younger in appearance and in activity by following the instructions in this book. Sid was a friend and became a patient only after the coronary thrombosis very nearly ended his life in his early thirties. He thought that he was in the best of good health since he played tennis regularly, occasionally enjoyed golf and even jogged. However, his general nutrition was so poor that his devitalized tissues could not take the degree of exercise or the degree of stress produced by that exercise as well as by his work. I explained to Sid that practically everybody is functioning below optimal capacity, which results from not eating properly. I told him everything that you have already learned through these consultations to this point and placed him on the Revitalization Cocktail containing the poly-unsaturated fat of safflower oil. I advised him to take 800 I.U. of vitamin E, five grams of vitamin C with his morning cocktail and another five grams to improve his immune system as well as many other functions of his body in another cocktail consisting simply of the vitamin C and orange juice in mid-afternoon or early evening. He, too, was placed on the half-portion diet, and he was to take sunflower seeds with his meals in the morning for their high vitamin and fiber content, as well as a high-dosage general vitamin and mineral supplement capsule or tablet. I also felt it important for him to have an additional capsule containing all of the known B-vitamins, which he was to take either at the same time or with lunch or dinner. I suggested two meals a day, no smoking (he had smoked one pack a day) and a limit to alcohol. Naturally, Sid was to avoid starch and sugar and generally to be on a high-fiber diet. Twenty years later, appearing twenty years younger than his age, he is back playing tennis, although I advised him to play only doubles and never to play to win, but only for the fun of it. He appears capable in every way and even learned to take the aggression out of his games. I have no doubt that he will live a long life, enjoy his restored youth and renewed vitality and probably never have a second "coronary."

††How to Do it Yourself.

1. **Begin your day with the Revitalization Cocktail. This is the natural route to a regularly emptied, completely and easily emptied bowel.**
2. **Your diet must be a half-portion diet, low in sugar and fats in order to stop and reverse the aging process in many of your cells, tissues and organs.**
3. **Practice the relaxation techniques you have learned throughout these consultations in order to empty your brain and be born anew each day. Do this each night of your life, for the next one-hundred years.**
4. **Avoid additives by avoiding processed foods, starches and sugars.**
5. **Drink large quantities of hard water. The minerals are of great importance to your arteries.**
6. **Remember that the less you eat, the longer you will live (assuming you are eating an optimal diet at an optimal weight).**

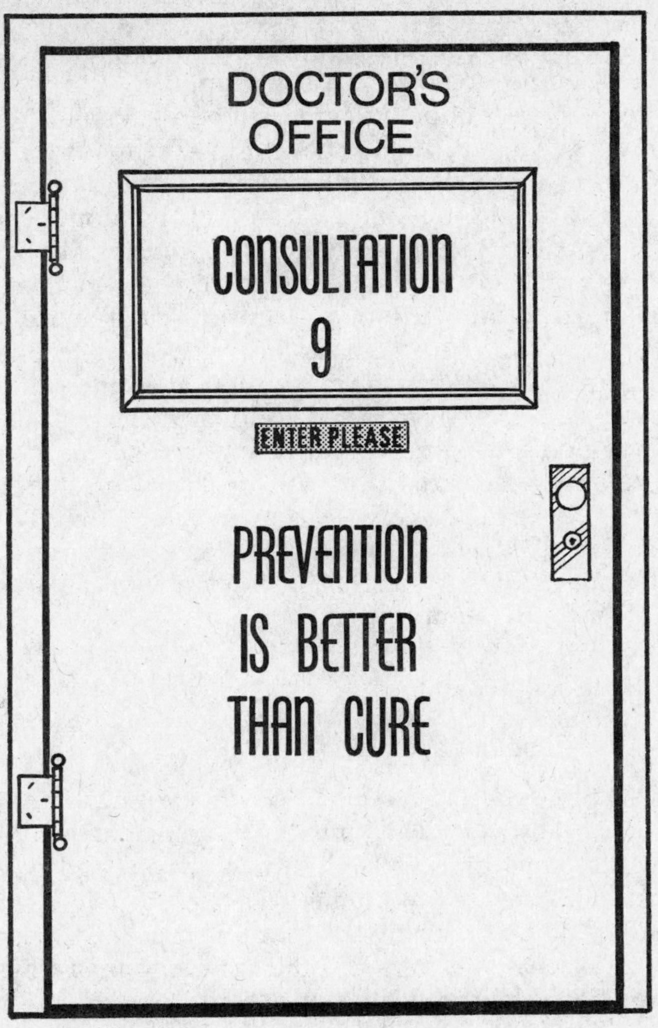

DOCTOR'S
OFFICE
CONSULTATION
9
ENTER PLEASE
PREVENTION
IS BETTER
THAN CURE

It must be obvious to you, now that we are at our ninth consultation, that the main purpose of this book is to teach you how to prevent disease. It may even be possible, under certain circumstances, and with the appropriate approach, to prevent or delay the development of cancer. It may become possible as well, to delay or prevent the formation of metastases after surgical removal of a primary cancer. Much important research is being done in this direction at the present time.

I have told you about such research by the National Cancer Institute in reference to a "cousin" of vitamin A. It is too early to say, but there is great hope that this will be a suitable and simple cancer preventive agent. Also, I have told you about the prolongation of life in otherwise rapidly terminal cancer patients as a result of simply taking 10 grams of vitamin C by mouth each day. That work was done in Scotland and is continuing. There is also evidence, as reported by a Japanese researcher, that vitamin C increases the development of the important T-lymphocytes. These lymphocytes are the warriors that fight—one-to-one—with developing cancer cells. If the T-lymphocytes are sufficient in number, the cancer may well be held in check.

We are interested in preventing the major killers of our day, cardiovascular disease and cancer. We are also interested, in these consultations, in learning how to prevent premature aging and early death. And finally, we wish to revitalize cells, tissues and organs that are in the process of self-destruction as a result of inadequate or improper nutrition.

And so, we come to the ancient conclusion that "Prevention is better than cure."

††*How Bill C. Conquered Asthma*

Bill C. had a serious problem. He was a youngster not yet 13 years of age when I was called into a conference on his problem. He had had asthma practically from infancy on, and despite all medications and the many eminent specialists who were consulted, the condition became worse each year. Finally, despite the fact that his parents had followed the instructions of physicians, and moved with their child to various sections of this country supposedly free from allergic pollens and such, the condition became desperate.

I received a telephone call asking if I knew any way to help. I indicated, of course, that without having the full previous history from his physicians and seeing the youngster at this time, there was obviously no advice I could give over the telephone. They told me that they had been informed of the books I had written on psychosomatic medicine and thought that perhaps the psychosomatic approach might be helpful to their son. Indeed, my name had been given to them by several physicians with that in mind.

They agreed to send him to New York, and when Bill entered my office it was as if a walking skeleton had brought the shadow of death into my consultation room. The boy was obviously in an almost terminal stage of depletion of his body structure, and he was naturally almost lethargic and depressed. A complete study by various physicians to whom I referred him, found no evidence of other disease, but all threw up their hands in a hopeless gesture of despair. They did not feel that anything more could be done for him.

I sent Bill back to his parents with my opinion. I told his parents that it was my opinion that the boy was allergic to them. I knew this was difficult for them to accept, but I asked them to accept it as a possibility since all other physicians had failed and no drugs were helpful. I told them of the Revitalization Plan and the Revitalization Cocktail, and I suggested that they send him to live somewhere apart from them; not in the same city, and preferably not in the same state. They were to be certain that wherever they boarded him, the instructions for proper nutrition were to be given to those who would care for him. They did this immediately, without question.

I am pleased to tell you that it is now almost 35 years since that occurred, and Bill is now the father of his own little family. He is a successful attorney and only has asthma when he visits his parents or his parents visit him. We see in this case the combination of psyche (mind) and soma (body) in the cause of a serious, sometimes fatal, always disabling disorder. We see the importance of treating the mind-body as a single unit. And, we see how the simple removal of the patient from a stressful environment, combined with appropriate nutrition to rebuild the body-mind, may save a life.

Preventive Power in Common Foods

What could be more "common" than orange juice? And yet, this common food contains true magic. Ascorbic acid, commonly known as vitamin C, is the source of that magic. When you add vitamin C crystals to juice, you produce what I call "fortified orange juice." I need not tell you about the tremendous power in fortified orange juice. Fortified orange juice, or fortified skimmed milk (produced in the same fashion by the addition of vitamin C), or fortified grapefruit juice (or any other juice you prefer), is a major factor in the Revitalization Cocktail.

And, during these consultations, I have told you about my use of sunflower seeds and skimmed milk cottage cheese as part of my own breakfast. The magic of sunflower seeds is extensive, and I need not repeat what you have already learned. I do hope that by this time your breakfast also contains several ounces of sunflower seeds, as well as the skimmed milk cottage cheese and the other ingredients of the Revitalization Cocktail.

Think of the amazing preventive power in soybeans. Turn back to Consultation 4, and read about the importance of the soybean that not only provides the best protein in the vegetable kingdom, but provides essential vitamins and minerals as well. This is indeed a magic natural package of energy. Add this energy to your nutritional intake and you will be revitalizing every cell, every tissue and every organ of your body.

I have told you about selenium in onions. Here we have another magic mineral that reverses the aging of heart and arteries by its action on cholesterol.

You have learned of the importance of vanadium in ocean fish, especially in the herring, which is also magic for the prevention and even the reversal of aging of the heart and arteries. Again, we have a mineral that acts to reduce cholesterol in the bloodstream.

The importance of natural, raw, unprocessed wheat germ bran is now known to you, and you are using it in your Revitalization Cocktail. Unprocessed, coarse wheat bran should be kept refrigerated so that it does not lose its nutritional power. It contains protein, carbohydrate, fat, vitamin A, vitamin C, (neither in very large quantity), thiamine, riboflavin, niacin, calcium and iron. The proportion of these latter minerals and vitamins range from approximately 10 percent of the USRDA in a two-ounce serving to as much as 50 percent for niacin and iron.

The brewer's type yeast, also very important in your Revitalization Cocktail, contains the excellent range of amino acids, such as alanine, aspartic acid, arginine, cystine, glutomic acid, glycine, histidine, hydroxyproline, isoleucine, leucine, lysine, methionine, phenylalanine, proline, threonine, tryptophane, tyrosine and valine. The essential amino acids in this group are histidine, isoleucine, leucine, lysine, methionine, phenylalanine, threonine, tryptophane and valine. The yeast that I use in my Revitalization Cocktail contains 50 percent protein. It also contains thiamine, riboflavin, niacin, vitamin B^6 and pantothenic acid. There are very tiny quantities of vitamin A and vitamin C as well.

The lecithin granules that I personally use are, of course, of soybean origin. They contain choline, inositol, phosphorus, and polyunsatured fatty acids (the important linoleic acid).

The preventive power in these common foods is now well known to you. It is obvious that if you drink your Revitalization Cocktail, and follow the Revitalization Plan of eating, you will have an adequate quantity of "preventive power" in those foods. But we go beyond that in terms of the total plan by adding a supplementary high-vitamin/high-mineral capsule or tablet, to be certain that you not only have a recommended daily allowance, but an *optimal* daily allowance.

††How Spencer R. Controlled Hypoglycemia and the Common Cold

I must begin by telling you that most doctors consider that hypoglycemia is either very uncommon or not even a "real" disease. There are some physicians who specialize, on the other hand, in the treatment of hypoglycemia, and believe that it is very common, but not easily recognized. I write of it here only in terms of what I have read in the literature and what I have been told by one of my patients, Spencer R. I do not treat hypoglycemia or diabetes. I believe that the treatment of such conditions should be under the care of the diabetologist. He is the best informed in the matter of blood sugar levels and the appropriate treatment for disorders of this nature. When I saw this patient he was consulting me for rectal bleeding, and I found small hemorrhoids which I treated by injection with a sclerosing solution. I advised him against surgery, especially since he was under treatment by the referring internist for "hypoglycemia."

Dr. Harvy M. Ross of California believes that as much as 10 percent of the population of the United States suffers from hypoglycemia. Assuming that is so, it is certainly worth considering this condition in a text on nutriton. To increase the importance of such consideration, there are claims that there is a close association between hypoglycemia and schizophrenia.

The patient with hypoglycemia has a low blood-sugar level after eating the easily absorbed processed carbohydrates such as sugar and white flour. Obviously, if you follow the Revitalization Plan, you will not be eating this type of sugar. That, in itself, could prevent hypoglycemia, and perhaps even be helpful—assuming the association claimed is correct—in the management of schizophrenia. The symptoms described by Spencer R. included a lack of energy, a feeling of faintness where he felt that he was ready to "fall to the ground," and insomnia. He tells me that other patients with his kind of condition, being treated by his internist, have headaches and pain in various parts of their bodies. He did not have such headaches or pain.

The diagnosis of hypoglycemia, of course, requires a careful study of blood sugar with a "five or six hour glucose-tolerance test." The fasting level is said to fall very low, as much as 60 milligrams percent.

The treatment recommended is to avoid processed carbohydrates and caffeine and to eat a low-carbohydrate, high-protein diet. Of course, if you are on the Revitalization Program you will be doing exactly that and more. In addition to preventing hypoglycemia, it is obvious that the Revitalization Plan goes far beyond this in terms of reenergizing, strengthening and revitalizing every cell, tissue and organ of your body insofar as they can be restored to optimal health.

Fortunately, Spencer was not subject to schizophrenia and had nothing to report on that from a personal level. Schizophrenics should really be under the care of a capable psychiatrist although it is obvious that good nutrition will be helpful in every type of disease.

Now, as for the common cold, I advised Spencer R. on the addition of 10 grams of vitamin C to his daily diet in conjunction with the Revitalization Cocktail, and six months later when he returned for reexamination of the rectum, I was pleased to advise him that he needed no further treatment. His hemorrhoids were now very small and no longer showed any evidence of bleeding. He, in turn, pleased me by telling me that since he had started with the Revitalization Cocktail with 10 grams of vitamin C each day, he ceased having the frequent colds which he had had in the past.

††*How Susan V. Overcame Constant Nausea*

Susan V., an attractive youngster of 32, had been suffering from practically constant nausea for the past eight months. She had visited a gastroenterologist and had been given a complete and thorough study by that specialist, who found no evidence of pathology. She had heard about the possibility of the condition being psychosomatic, had asked the gastroenterologist about that and was told to consult a psychiatrist or a psychologist. He indicated that it might indeed be the result of an emotional disturbance.

As I recall, it was through a former patient that Susan V. became aware of the fact that I had written extensively on that subject and came to me for consultation. She had followed the instructions of her gastroenterologist very carefully and had taken the various medications he prescribed, all to no avail. In the early stages, she thought that perhaps she was "pregnant," since she lived an open sex life. It became obvious, with the passage of time, that she was not pregnant. Susan told me that although she felt she was a liberated woman, she really did not enjoy her liberation very much. She did enjoy her work as an expert stenotypist, working for a firm that specialized in legal cases.

I questioned Susan V. carefully on the matter of diet and asked that she make a list of everything she ate and the time that she did the eating for an entire week, and then return to me with that list. She did and I was astonished to find that her diet was chiefly Coca-cola, Pesi cola, sandwiches and coffee. The very thought of living only on these foods was enough to give me a sense of nausea.

I promptly started her on the Revitalization Cocktail and the entire program. At first, she told me that the cocktail itself nauseated her. After a time, however, she came to enjoy it and recognized that she was feeling much healthier, much stronger, slept better and was much happier as she became accustomed to the cocktail and the entire program. The nausea ended, and Susan V. developed a new outlook on life. Without her nausea she lost her fear of pregnancy and began to enjoy a normal sex life with a young man whom she ultimately married.

Medicines from "Nature's Kitchen"

It must be obvious to you now that the best medicines do not come from the physician's prescription, nor from the drug store. They are readily available in what I call "nature's kitchen." Let us consider the soybean for example. Soybeans offer one of the cheapest forms of very nutritious protein. It will cost you pennies rather than dollars if you buy dried soybeans in a sufficient quantity to serve four persons. You will be providing protein quality that is the equivalent of meat or fish at a minor fraction of the price. You already know (see Consultation 4) about the general importance of the soybean and the precise content of soybeans in terms of vitamins and the very important unsaturated fatty acids, especially lecithin. There is little starch in soybeans, and they fit well into the best type of "medicine" from "nature's kitchen."

Soymilk was developed by Dr. Harry W. Miller, which is a lifesaver for babies who cannot use ordinary milk. Adults may also be allergic to cow's milk, and soymilk is a perfect replacement. You can use soymilk as the base for your Revitalization Cocktail in place of skimmed milk or fruit juice.

In China, soybean curd is called "the meat without the bone." I suggest that you find a recipe book on the use of the soybean. You will be astonished at how much you can do with soybeans at little cost and with the finest nutrition. The concentrated protein that is in soybeans as "soyflour" offers a perfect protein for everyone, again at a low price. It is also rich in phosphorus, calcium, iron ,riboflavin, thaimine and niacin as well as many minerals, such as copper, magnesium and iron. You can also obtain a soyflour that contains lecithin as well.

"Nature's kitchen" also provides us with a tremendous assortment of fresh fruits and vegetables. Whenever possible, eat your fruits and vegetables without cooking. If you must cook them, do not cook them long and try a pressure cooker. You will then have reserved for your own nutrition the best qualities of the food, and will lose little of it to the cooking device. Safflower oil, sunflower seed oil, the sunflower seeds themselves and all types of nuts, offer high quality foods from "nature's kitchen." You will be using the sunflower seeds and the safflower oil in your own kitchen to revitalize your body. Indeed, wherever possible, try to avoid commercial foods, and foods that do not come from "nature's kitchen." You will be healthier, and you will live longer.

††*How Richard Y. Overcame Acid Indigestion and Escaped Ulcer Surgery*

I saw this patient after he had been advised to have surgery for a duodenal ulcer. There was no doubt that Richard Y. did have a duodenal ulcer, but there was also no doubt that he had been eating a very unhealthful diet and had been living a very stressful life. He was important in an advertising agency, but saw no possibility of getting close to the "top." The stress and anxiety resulting from this desire to be the "top dog" in his agency was giving him acid indigestion. The types of luncheons and dinners that he was forced to "enjoy" with the prospective customers for the agency were also giving him acid indigestion. The final result was a clearly visible ulcer of the small intestine directly following the outlet of the stomach (the duodenum).

Richard Y. had not been helped by the treatment offered by his gastroenterologist, perhaps because that treatment consisted almost entirely of the use of antacids. Such drugs sometimes have a so-called "rebound effect," causing still more acid to form after the initial relief produced by the antacid. His diet had been properly modified in terms of the gastroenterologist's suggestions, but neither the antacids nor the prescribed diet seemed to have helped. Subsequently, he was ordered to go under the surgeon's knife.

I told him that such ulcers could perforate or hemorrhage and that he really should follow the advice of the gastroenterologist and the surgeon. He rebelled and said that he would rather die. Indeed, he felt that he would die on the operating table. He begged me to do what I could for him with diet alone.

I warned Richard Y. that diet alone could not be the final answer for him, since his work was so stressful. Unless he changed his attitude toward work, gave up the driving desire to be "top dog" in his agency and become more relaxed in his daily life, diet alone would probably not be very helpful. Richard realized the truth of what I was saying and agreed to try but did not seem very hopeful. I put him on the Revitalization Plan formulas and taught him how to meditate and how to relax. He was a very apt student.

I advised him that he could only live one day at a time, one moment at a time, one heartbeat at a time, and if he preferred to devote those moments and those heartbeats to chasing the position of top executive in his organization and adding more money to his bank account, the best he could hope for would be ultimate surgery and a larger bank account. If that is what he wanted, that is what he would have.

In time, Richard became very adept at relaxation, practiced the meditation formulas several times a day, changed his diet completely (even during business luncheons) to fit into the plan I had outlined and learned to take each moment, each hour and each day "in stride." The results were excellent. Within three months, the acid indigestion had ended and a repeat X-ray study showed improvement in the extent of the duodenal ulcer. Richard Y. stayed with his routine, with the approval of his gastroenterologist, and after the first fourteen months, no further sign of the ulcer could be found on the X-ray study.

I must caution you that this is an exceptional result. Only a very intelligent, very cooperative individual, strongly opposed to surgery, could attempt this approach in the face of the specialist's advice to have a surgical removal of the ulcer area. However, the total mind-body approach should be used even if surgery is performed. It is important to relieve these patients from stress as well as from the damage produced by an ulcer.

††*Your Instructions for Today. . .*

1. **Eat only the foods from "nature's kitchen," and avoid food with additives, high starch content and high sugar content of the supermarket variety.**
2. **If you are told that you have hypoglycemia you may wish to try the Revitalization Plan diet. It is the precise diet that is offered by those doctors who claim to see many such cases.**
3. **To overcome nausea and to aid in the relief, prevention and perhaps cure of peptic ulcer, you should give a fair trial to the Revitalization Cocktail and the Revitalization Plan. Remain under the careful observation of your personal physician during this time, and follow his advice.**

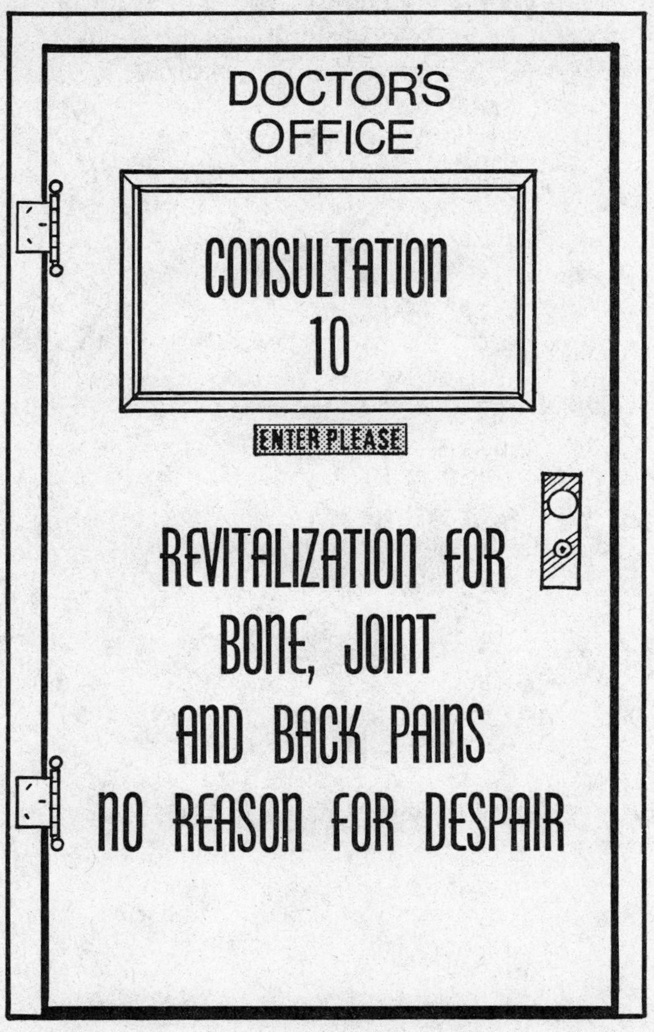

You may be experiencing pain and painful spasms in the various muscles and joints of your body, such that you can no longer move your legs or arms freely. This is common in people who are aging prematurely. Back pain and back stiffness are, of course, extremely common, and all of these conditions are associated with muscle spasm. Then there are those who complain of general aches and pains; some use the word "neuritis" to describe their pain. Obviously, we are talking about many different problems with similiar symptoms. Sometimes the symptoms are so severe that the patient is disabled. Arthritis, of course, is a chronic disease, a serious crippler, and unfortunately, we do not have specific answers to the arthritis problem.

But, don't despair! With proper diet and exercise and adequate supervision by your physician, most of these symptoms can be controlled, even though the basic underlying disease is not well understood. If you can find a specialist to assist you in your treatment, please do so. For our own purposes during these consultations, I suggest that a basic need for all such patients is the Revitalization Program. This program will supply the best possible nutrients to protect every cell, tissue and organ of the body and to stimulate your defenses against bone, joint and back pain problems.

Always bear in mind that it is important that you should not allow a joint to become stiff by neglect. If you sit motionless for most of the day, these stiff joints will become relatively fixed in position and may require surgery.

However, if you practice the Buddha Walk and Buddha Dance each day, never forcing the stiff muscles, bone or joint beyond the point of excess pain, you will find in many cases that the range of motion will increase and the pain will be relieved. This is not a "cure." But, since there is no known cure for arthritis and since regular exercise each day of the measured type described in these consultations will help you to increase the range of motion in the distressed joints, do not fail to perform these exercises as often as you can throughout the day. If your physician approves, he may also want you to try aspirin in moderate dosage to help relieve discomfort.

I have already described the simple and pleasant exercise of pretending that you are leading an orchestra. Do this while listening to your favorite music and you will find that stiff muscles, stiff joints, muscle spasm discomfort in your arms, forearms and shoulders will gradually improve and may allow an increased range of motion when the tight or tense muscles are released. Fear of motion and fear of pain are factors that will be put to rest as you gradually develop your capacity for leading the orchestra as in Consultation 6.

There are those who believe niacinamide in large dosage (1-4 grams daily) will relieve the pain of arthritis and improve the range of motion in stiff joints. I have spoken of this in Consultation 1 and have nothing to add at this point. Certainly, there is no objection to trying this vitamin.

There are also those who claim that very large dosages of vitamin C will help in controlling arthritis symptoms. The dosage described is often so high that it must certainly be given under the proper supervision of a surgeon, orthopedist or, perhaps, a nutritionist. I have no experience with the enormous dosage of vitamin C recommended for this problem and certainly make no claims for its value.

What is Rheumatism?

Many patients speak of having "rheumatism" when they experience the type of symptoms we have been describing, including practically all types of pains and aches in joints, muscles and so on. The word has been misused so often that it really has no specific meaning.

In the past, treatment for "rheumatism" was to remove focal infection. This resulted in extensive surgery of all types, from tonsils and adenoids to internal organs such as the appendix, the gallbladder and sometimes even segments of the large bowel. It is hard to believe in the present state of the art of medicine that this was once the commonly accepted medical practice. Obviously, if you have this type of symptom your best bet is to follow the Revitalization Program. Certainly, you do not need surgery. On the other hand, when there is a seriously diseased organ or tissue, it should be properly treated, and that is where your personal physician can help you.

What About Arthritis?

I believe I have pretty much covered the subject in our sixth consultation. Regrettably there is no specific treatment for arthritis. Beware of new "wonder drugs." Once again, I recommend the various exercises described in the Revitalization Program and, of course, the basic diet. Practice muscle-relaxing as described throughout these consultations. For discomfort, aspirin is perhaps at least as effective as any other medicine and certainly much less expensive. It is here that your family physician can best advise you.

If you surrender to the arthritis you will become progressively more crippled. If you retain hope and an optimistic attitude toward life and if you follow the Revitalization Program in all its aspects, you will certainly improve your general health, and this offers the best possible basis for healthier muscles, bones and joints.

††*The Case of Arthur S.*

Arthur S. consulted me at 32 years of age because of ulcerative colitis. He also had asthma attacks in his childhood, but had "outgrown" these.

His history included many stress factors. As an actor, he was often either out of work and out of money or heavily in debt to friends. He had become more successful of late and he was working regularly at the time that he consulted me.

However, his emotional tensions stayed with him, and these tensions reflected themselves in limited motion of the joints and stiffness of the muscles.

I taught Arthur the Buddha Walk and the Buddha Dance. He liked the concept of "leading an orchestra" to music in his own home, and he practiced these exercises regularly.

I also taught him how to relax all the muscles of his body so that he would more easily achieve direct control of the stiffness in the painful muscles and joints. When he "relaxed to the point of sleep," as he put it, he found that he could very gradually increase the range of motions in each of the involved joints without pain.

With walking, I told Arthur to use the self-suggestion of, "Every day, in every way, my muscles and joints are becoming healthier and healthier, stronger and stronger, younger and younger."

This type of positive reprogramming of the stress-filled mind is very effective. It should be used at every possible opportunity, not only while practicing relaxation or the various exercises of the Revitalization Program, but even while working, eating and at bedtime. The bedtime programming is the best of all.

I am pleased to report that Arthur improved greatly while using the total Revitalization Program, with special emphasis upon the above techniques. When he departed New York for the West Coast to continue his increasingly active acting career, he was in much better health and spirits and proved to be very successful in motion pictures.

So, we see that stress, disturbed life patterns, financial, physical and emotional problems, in a word, "environmental stress" from childhood on may be basic in causing bone, joint and back pains. If you feel that there is a strong emotional background for your own problem, consult with your physician and have him refer you to a qualified psychiatrist or psychologist. But, always remember that the emotions are only one factor in the total picture. However, they may be the major underlying factor that ultimately destroys the body's defense in the involved areas. Once again, your best bet is the total Revitalization Program so that you will be providing the proper nutrition as well as the proper mental-emotional environment for the disturbed bones, joints or back problems.

Arthritis and Niacinamide

Many years ago, I called together some of the outstanding physicians in psychiatry, surgery, general medicine and other limited specialties, with the emphasis upon psychology and psychiatry, and we met at the Waldorf Hotel in New York. I had written to each, informing them that my plan was to establish a new society, the Academy of Psychosomatic Medicine, to bring the insights of the psychiatrists and psychologists to the average physician. This would enable all physicians to understand the psychosomatic concept and the importance of treating the entire patient—the "mind-body" as I put it—rather than simply a sore throat, hemorrhoids, cancer and so forth.

This society now boasts a membership of three thousand, and I am proud to have been its founder and am currently President Emeritus.

One of the men I called to this first organizational meeting was a Dr. William Kaufman, who practiced in the New England area. He is now retired, but has remained active in related areas of medicine. Dr. Kaufman studied and treated patients with many disorders but was especially interested in joint problems such as limitation of motion and arthritis.

He dispensed his own medications and recommended large, mega doses of niacinamide from 400 mg. to over 2200 mg. for joint dysfunctions. He claimed that the results were good in improving the range of motion of the involved joint, but agreed that there might well be a placebo effect as well. The "powerful" placebo is an inert substance—the sugar coated inert pill—that so impresses the patient (together with the physician's reputation or mystique), that the patient feels better even though the "pill" has no chemical or other pharmacological effect.

I do not know of anyone who now prescribes large dosages of niacinamide for arthritis, but Dr. Linus Pauling, the famous Nobel Laureate in chemistry, has advised me in a personal communication that a close member of his family with arthritis has indeed benefited from one or two grams of niacinamide as a daily dose.

He advised me that Doctor A. (please see Consultation 1), who had developed a migratory arthralgia after taking large doses of vitamin A over a long period of time in an effort to control further development of cancer, might well benefit by taking one to four grams of niacinamide daily. He based his opinion primarily on the writings of Dr. Kaufman.

I passed along this information to Dr. A., who still has some residual arthralgia, and limited motion in the ring finger of his right hand, and he is now experimenting with one gram of niacinamide each day. He is, of course, also continuing with vitamin A in a decreased dose of 10,000 I.U. daily, plus whatever amount there might be in his carrot juice and vitamin C cocktail each day. It is too early to report complete results, although the residual arthralgia seems resistant to the niacinamide.

Total Program Therapy

In my opinion, until the day when a specific medication is discovered for arthritis, the total Revitalization Program is your best bet. I have no objection to a trial of niacinamide, say one gram a day to start, but as I have said elsewhere in this book, I know of no specific treatment or drug for arthritis.

I urge you, if this is your problem, to follow the dietary program I have outlined for you. I also suggest that you practice the Buddha Walk and the Buddha Dance to the limits of your joint range and function each day, or even several times a day if you can.

I also urge that you practice the exercise of leading an orchestra. I know of no concert orchestra conductor who has died young. Leopold Stokowski recently passed away quietly in his sleep; he was in his mid-nineties. The exercise and the power of the music to quiet the mind and concentrate it away from the troubles and cares of the day will aid you in letting go. When you "let go" you will find the stiffness decreasing, the discomfort disappearing and an increased range of motion.

††*Your Prescriptions for Today...*

1. **Stay away from those who promise "cure," since there is no specific remedy for arthritis.**
2. **If you have not already done so, begin the Revitalization Program at once. Do not stray from the total pattern of that program.**
3. **Give special attention to the Buddha Walk and the Buddha Dance, and learn to "lead your own orchestra."**
4. **Practice relaxation and reprogramming of your body-mind throughout the day, especially before you go to sleep each night.**

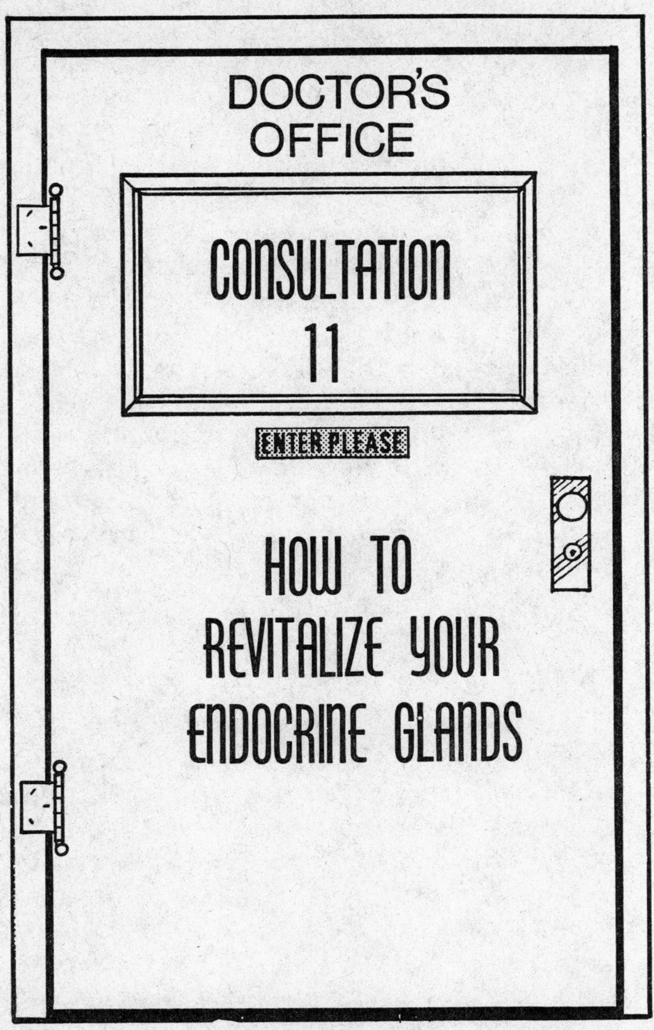

DOCTOR'S
OFFICE
CONSULTATION
11
ENTER PLEASE
HOW TO
REVITALIZE YOUR
ENDOCRINE GLANDS

How to Recognize An Endocrine Problem

You have already learned a great deal about the endocrine glands throughout these consultations. I have told you about the powerful pituitary gland at the base of the brain, the master gland that controls all the others. In our consultations, you will find important data on the relationship between the thalamus, the hypothalamus and the pituitary gland. The thalamus and hypothalamus are located at the base of the brain, and they seem to mediate stress and other emotions, partially through the pituitary gland and from there to all parts of the body.

So, if you are overly emotional, excitable or jittery, there may be an endocrine problem or an endocrine-mediated problem. If your appetite is poor or if you are losing weight rapidly while eating well, we may again be dealing with an endocrine problem. If you eat relatively a small amount but are still gaining weight, or have a ravenous appetite, this may also be related to a dysfunction of your endocrine glands. I have seen many patients who are depressed easily, and although this may be due to stress, anxieties about the future or constant reliving of the problems of the past, such depression can be endocrine mediated.

The physician can readily recognize a possible endocrine problem if he notes that your eyes protrude in a glassy stare. Or, if you are a woman, perhaps your monthly periods are not regular. The possibility of diabetes may come to your physician's attention when you tell him that you are always hungry, always thirsty and urinate a great deal.

††*The Case of Mrs. R.*

When Mrs. R. consulted me, she told me that she had been on the verge of a nervous breakdown several times throughout her marriage and even before that when her mother died. She thought that her intended marriage to a man that her mother did not consider worthy of her, might have "broken her heart" and she felt that she was responsible for her mother's death.

Mrs. R. married at 18 years of age, and when I saw her at 33 she had two children. Her husband was twelve years older than she, and she had been in High School at the time of her marriage. It was obvious that she had married as a rebellion against her parents. She told me that she "could not stand the constant fighting over money, and wanted to have a husband who could support her without any problems."

Her husband was a complete disappointment to her sexually. He did support her well, but "he was not exactly my idea of what marriage should be like." A husband who came home after a hard day's work, "plopped in front of a television set with a bottle of beer and then fell asleep," was not what she expected of marriage. Mrs. R. never had an orgasm, and sex was a total disappointment to her. She had been to physicians who had offered to instruct her husband in sex matters, but they had not been successful. She finally decided to abandon this approach.

She had moderate finger tremor, wet palms and a flush of the neck and lower face, all of which indicate a possible thyroid overactivity. An appropriate blood test of the protein-bound iodine indicated a mild thyroid overactivity.

What this patient needed was explanation, reassurance and finally, by her own choice, a new life with a still older man after divorcing her husband. I placed Mrs. R. on the Revitalization Program, and she found great release from stress and anxiety when she practiced the Buddha Walk, the Buddha Dance and the relaxation technique before going to sleep.

Your Emotions and Your Thyroid

Some thyroid anxiety problems are sufficiently severe to require treatment with radioactive iodine or even partial removal of the thyroid. It is important that adequate nutrition and appropriate psychotherapy be continued throughout the medical or surgical treatment, and in some cases for a lifetime.

Emotional disturbances are always part of thyroid problems. They may be the cause or the effect. When thyroid overactivity is controlled by medications or surgery, the emotional problems may disappear. If they do not, you must consult a trained psychologist or psychiatrist. An emotional shock is very often followed by a serious thyroid imbalance—a toxic thyroid. However, it is very difficult to distinguish ordinary anxiety symptoms from early overactivity of the thyroid gland. Look for the sweating palm, the flushing neck, the slight tremor of the fingertips when the hands are extended. These are telltale signs.

Very often, there has been a severe emotional problem just before these thyroid symptoms begin. You cannot treat such conditions yourself, and if you seek to avoid the problem by running away from it, you will be making a mistake. Always consult your physician, have the necessary studies done and then follow his advice. You may need a psychologist, a psychiatrist and possibly a surgeon. You will also need to follow the Revitalization Program in order to provide the best possible nutrition for your entire body, including your endocrine glands.

††*The Case of Lazy Thyroid*

I remember a patient whom I saw in 1964, a Mrs. R. L. She was 32 years old at that time and told me that she had "always been fat." I advised her that she should lose about 50 pounds in order to conform her body structure, height and weight to the norms of the best-weight tables.

She came from a family that ate large meals at least three times a day and often ate in-between. Her mother believed that unless she ate well she would not "be well." The quality of food was good, with the exception that there was considerable stress on fatty meats and an enormous quantity of food. The result was a family of seriously overweight individuals.

The protein-bound iodine test of her blood evidenced a sluggish thyroid. Mrs. R.L. had already been treated for obesity by many so-called "specialists" who had given her a great variety of pills. Obviously, some of these pills contained large amounts of amphetamines, and when I finally saw her, she was literally "hooked" on these drugs. The result was that she could not sleep at night and was jittery all day.

When placed on the Revitalization Diet, together with the thyroid analog pills to reinforce her lazy thyroid, she lost weight without the premature wrinkling and aging that often accompanies a rapid weight loss. Of great importance to her was the half-portion idea as well as the total nutrient program of the Revitalization concept.

The lazy thyroid condition is very common. If you are overweight, do consult your physician for an appropriate thyroid test and follow his instructions. The protein-bound iodine test is very simple and requires only a small blood sample from an arm vein. I believe it to be more reliable than the basal-metabolism test.

††*The Interesting Case of Joan L.*

A few years before seeing the above case, I had treated an eighteen year old youngster who was 31 pounds overweight. Joan L. complained of being constantly tired, and she preferred to sleep rather than be awake. Since Joan was not only 31 pounds overweight but was also "always unhappy," it was obvious that we had a serious emotional-endocrine problem.

Joan's parents had taken her to many doctors and she told them that she did not eat very much. However, she complained, "nobody believes me."

I did believe her. Her problem was a lazy thyroid, and her retreat from reality was due to the combination of the lazy thyroid and the emotional problems of school as well as at home.

The treatment was the Revitalization Diet combined with the thyroid analog pills. Fortunately, Joan L. responded well and did not need further treatment by a psychologist or a psychiatrist.

Anorexia Nervosa

Anorexia nervosa simply means nervous loss of appetite. This condition is seen chiefly in adolescent girls whose personality problem is that they are perfectionists; they have been given strict toilet training and are usually repelled by sex. They rarely masturbate, which is usually a very normal thing to do.

I mention this condition here only because it may be confused with a pituitary-like dysfunction. In spite of eating well, such patients often continue to lose weight. Menstrual periods may stop, or there may be only a slight staining at monthly intervals. However, a complete examination will show nothing particularly unusual in such cases. Nevertheless, the weight loss may continue, and the problem then requires careful study by a physician and perhaps by an endocrinologist. Care by a psychologist or psychiatrist may also be indicated. Once the problem is resolved, these patients respond well to the Revitalization Program and lead a normal healthy life.

Revitalization Starts at Birth

It should be obvious to you now that proper diet must begin at birth. Actually, it should begin in terms of the best possible diet—The Revitalization Diet—for the mother during pregnancy. Modern obstetricians are now well aware of the importance of proper diet for the pregnant female. Without proper diet during that important time, the embryo may not develop normally, may be born with a serious defect and may not even survive the delivery.

I have often made the statement that we begin to die as soon as we are born—all of us. To postpone premature aging and early death, proper nutrition in infancy and childhood, proper emotional conditioning and the initiation of the total Revitalization Program as soon as possible must be assured. Your endocrine glands—and every cell, every tissue and every organ of your body—must be provided with the proper nutrients while in your mother's womb and afterwards.

Most of the readers of these consultations will not have had this advantage. Therefore, it becomes even more important that they be adequately instructed in terms of the Revitalization Program at the earliest possible date. If you wish to halt the process of dying that begins at birth you must start right now.

Mind-Body Control of the Endocrine Glands

The thalamus and hypothalamus sections of the brain, located at the base of the brain, are intimately related to our emotions and to the functions of the master gland, the pituitary gland. It becomes obvious, therefore, that you must learn to control your emotions if you are to avoid overactivity or underactivity of the master gland and all the other endocrine glands that are controlled by the master pituitary gland.

Once again, since you cannot do very much about the repressed emotional dynamite of your past, aside from consulting a psychiatrist or a psychologist, the mind-body elements of the total Revitalization Program should be put into action at the earliest possible date. Once again, this means *right now* for you.

Learn how to relax, practice the Buddha Walk and the Buddha Dance, accompanied by the proper reconditioning statement, "healthier and healthier, better and better, younger and younger," during the time that you are walking or dancing. You will find full instructions on this approach in the related consultations.

When you have learned to relax, to set a limit to your desires, to stop reliving the problem past, and to discontinue living in fear of the future, your body-mind will no longer be disarranged by an overactive endocrine system. In this way, you may prevent or rid yourself of psychosomatic health problems.

Low Blood-Sugar

My wife has experienced the low blood-sugar syndrome quite often. We would be walking down the street when she would say to me, "I am going to pass out." She would become faint, and we would have to find some place for her to obtain food. After several such experiences, it became evident that we were dealing with a functional hyperinsulinism, a condition in which her body seemed to produce too much insulin. She began to carry cheese or peanuts with her, which has helped to correct the condition.

Such rapid swings of the blood-sugar below the normal levels can leave any one of us easily fatigued, weak, or faint. Some of us develop such low blood-sugar levels because we drink too much coffee and suffer too much anxiety. Obviously, a physician must be consulted to be certain that there is no tumor of the pancreas. Such a tumor can produce excess insulin and cause precisely the same symptoms.

A major cause of these sudden swings of blood-sugar is anxiety, stress and improper diet. I must confess that it was only recently that my wife entered upon the complete Revitalization Program. Prior to that, she went from doctor to doctor, obviously not trusting someone as close as a husband. She was given many incorrect diagnoses, including diabetes.

A renowned diabetologist told my wife that she did not have diabetes (even though she had a family history of that condition) and that there was no such thing as hypoglycemia. He was, perhaps, right with regard to *his* definition of hypoglycemia, but to me it simply meant a case of low blood-sugar. It seemed to me quite obvious that she did have low blood-sugar during the times she was faint and easily fatigued. Stress, anxiety and worry about the past and the future were the answer, or cause, in her case.

Selye and Stress

The total Revitalization Program is the best way to approach stress, since it takes into account the mind as well as the body, the emotions and the anxiety that all of us suffer in one fashion or another, at one time or another.

My good friend, Dr. Hans Selye of Montreal, the most famous authority on stress research, has informed us that we all react to stress in very much the same fashion. He called this reaction "the general adaptation syndrome." But when the adaptation fails, for one reason or another, we can develop diseases, or in other words, health problems based on body-mind dysfunction.

Selye correctly pointed out that stress causes toxic substances to be released, and these substances then stimulate the endocrine glands, particularly the pituitary gland, to discharge a certain hormone which acts on our adrenal glands. These glands (which lie one on top of each kidney) then produce special hormones that increase and improve our resistance. This, in turn, reverses the changes in the various body tissues and organs and if the process has not gone on too long, we recover. But, when the stress continues and if we do not provide proper nutrients for the body-mind, we will once again become worse and may even die. Premature aging and premature death are the end result of continuous, unrelenting stress.

The Revitalization Program will reduce the likelihood of your ever developing high blood pressure, hardening of the arteries, coronary thrombosis or heart failure, arthritis and other debilitating ailments, and will increase your chances for better health and longer life.

What About Diabetes?

There seems to be an inherited deficiency in the pancreas so that it cannot produce sufficient insulin in those patients who develop diabetes. However, stress may precipate the first episode of diabetes. I remember one report from the Menninger Clinic on thirty mental disturbances in diabetics. The report was interesting primarily because when the "mental condition improved" these diabetics also improved without insulin and without dietary treatment. Appropriate psychotherapy made it possible for their blood-sugar levels to return to normal and for these patients to once again properly use sugar. These were depressed, anxious, neurotic people. Each emotional crisis set off an attack of "diabetes."

I remember seeing one such patient in 1960, a young man 34 years of age who had no interest in the opposite sex. This seemed to be a male-female hormonal imbalance, and he lived at home with his mother after his father died. He had indeed "hated" his father. His complaint was chronic fatigue. Although he was a noted interior decorator who enjoyed his work, he told me that life was "getting to be too much." His depression was such that he wished "to wake up dead."

The elevated blood sugar, spilling sugar into the urine, indicated after careful general study that he was indeed diabetic. There was no family history of disease in this case, and it was probably an emotionally triggered condition to a great extent.

We often discussed the value of life. We finally came to the obvious conclusion that there was nothing better either of us had to offer, and we might as well make the best of what we had. I pointed out to him, also, that he was making a contribution to the happiness of others by his excellence in his profession.

I placed him under the care of a diabetologist and he improved rapidly. He followed all the other elements of the Revitalization Program and has continued in an active, apparently productive and happy life.

††*Your Prescriptions for Today*

1. **Be kind to your endocrine glands, since they control how long you will live and whether or not you will age prematurely.**
2. **Provide your body with the total Revitalization Program.**

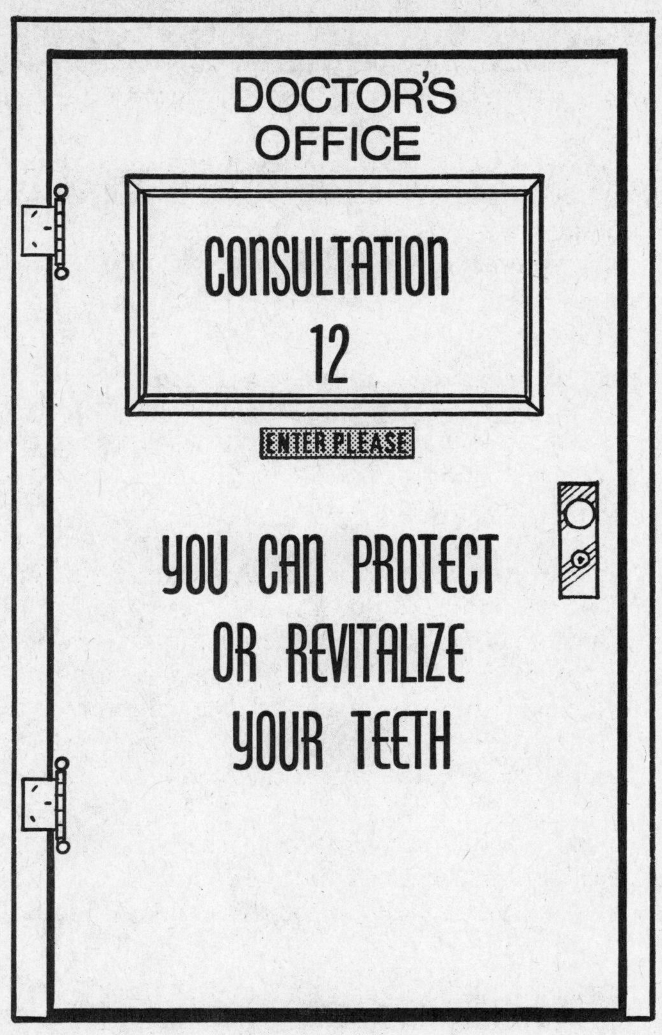

General Care

You should consult your dentist and ask him how to use dental floss, how to brush your teeth and massage your gums and how to remove tartar deposits in their earliest stages. You can easily do all of these relatively simple things as part of the daily home care of your teeth.

Prevention is always the better part of cure. The simple procedures your dentist advises will be the best part of local care and prevention, but the basic factor in prevention of decay and early loss of teeth rests with proper nutrition. If you provide your teeth with the proper nutrients as described in this book, especially calcium and phosphorus, the living teeth will retain their health and you may never enter the denture stage. Your teeth are set in bone, and the bones need proper nutrients in order to maintain their youthful composition and strength and to hold your teeth firmly in place.

How to Provide Basic Dental Nutrients

Quite simply; if you follow the Revitalization Program diet instructions you will automatically be offering your teeth and gums, as well as the bone structure in which your teeth are set, the best possible nutrition.

I have already mentioned calcium and phosphorus and must now add vitamin D to the list. But, the list does not end with these essential components. It must include all the factors of the Revitalization Program diet, since the teeth are dependent upon the living tissue components in the periodontal membrane and the pulp as well as in the bone and gums. If these surrounding and supporting tissues are not healthy, your teeth will soon decay and be lost.

You should also have fluoride in your water supply. Many dental preparations also contain fluoride. Here, your dentist is your best friend, for he can advise you if you need special fluoride treatment.

Avoid sugar in any but its natural forms in fruits. Do not eat candy, cookies, cake, or drink sugar-filled commercial preparations. There seems to be no question that such sugar will hasten decay of your teeth. Certainly, it will endanger your general body health as well.

Finally, a word about the special importance of vitamin C. This vitamin is essential to the formation of collagen, the connective tissue substance that holds your body together.

I personally take twelve grams each day, as does Dr. Linus Pauling, the noted Nobel Laureate chemist. He has advised me, through personal communication, to use the mixed crystals of sodium ascorbate and ascorbic acid to avoid the acidity effect of ordinary vitamin C preparations (ascorbic acid alone) and to reduce the possibility of kidney-stone formation and irritation of the urinary surfaces during urination. Sodium ascorbate and ascorbic acid are simply two forms of the same vitamin—vitamin C, the first being basic and the second acid, thus counteracting each other to form a more neutral and less irritating vitamin C.

I take four grams in the morning in the Revitalization Cocktail, another four grams in the afternoon, after lunch, simply mixed into orange juice and a third four-gram amount in the evening, mixed into a glass of freshly made carrot juice (full of both vitamin C and selenium as well as vitamin A). Sometimes, I reverse this by taking the carrot juice combination after lunch rather than in the evening.

The Controversial Vitamin C

Throughout these consultations I have given you my opinion of the value of large amounts of vitamin C in your daily nutrition. I have described the dosage that I myself take, 12 grams a day in three divided doses, 4 grams after each meal.

The human body, in contrast to many other forms of animal life, cannot manufacture vitamin C. Indeed, regardless of how much we take, only a relatively small amount of the vitamin can be stored in the body since it is immediately used by the body tissues. There is, however, some storage in some of the body's endocrine glands, especially the important stress-reaction glands on the top of each kidney, the adrenal glands. The excess amount, not needed by the body, is excreted by the kidneys or exhaled by the lungs in the form of carbon dioxide.

Although it is known that vitamin C is essential to the human body, as it is in other animal tissue, very few recognize its extensive importance in maintaining good health. The connective tissue that holds the body together, collagen, which is also found in skin, bones and tendons, depends upon vitamin C for its formation. Carbohydrates cannot be properly utilized by the body without vitamin C. Our teeth and our bones require vitamin C for calcification and the growth of the cells in those tissues and others, such as osteoblasts, odontoblasts and fibroblasts. Finally, without vitamin C, the body cannot adequately absorb iron from the intestines for storage in the liver.

Vitamin C came into prominence when it was recognized that it was essential to have a small amount of vitamin C in the body in order to prevent scurvy. Today, with the ready availability of orange juice and a relatively well-balanced diet, you will certainly obtain sufficient vitamin C to prevent scurvy. On the other hand, there is the possibility that you may need larger amounts if your body is under stress or threatened by infection. It is difficult to produce evidence to this effect, but the supposition must be considered.

As for the use of vitamin C in massive dosage to protect against the common cold, I can only speak from my own experience. Since the time I have been taking 12 grams daily, I have not had a single cold. This does not mean that it will work similarly for others.

The eminent nutritionist, Dr. Jean Mayer (formerly Professor of Nutrition at Harvard University–1950 to 1976), believes that a toxic level is between two and four grams. He also states that the body's use of copper and vitamin B^{12} is seriously interfered with by a large dosage of vitamin C. Another problem he points out is the possibility of a loss of calcium in the bones, especially in the case of older women, due to a mega dosage of vitamin C. And finally, he speaks of the possibility of the formation of small kidney stones (gravel) in those who are prone to such formation, again as a result of a two to four gram intake of vitamin C.

Dr. Linus Pauling disputes these claims and recommends large dosage of vitamin C, not only for the common cold, but for the control of influenza and viral as well as bacterial diseases including hepatitis, poliomyelitis, viral pneumonia, measles, mumps, tuberculosis, chicken pox, shingles, viral meningitis and viral orchitis as well as the less deadly cold sores, canker sores and fever blisters. He also states that warts may disappear when treated with a salve containing ascorbic acid.

In his interesting book, *Vitamin C, The Common Cold and The Flu,* he reports that five to 10 grams of vitamin C each day will increase the formation of new lymphocyte cells, a very important factor in the treatment of infections and cancer.

These are extensive and important claims, and I can take no side in this argument other than to tell you of my personal experiences throughout these consultations and to advise you that I myself take 12 grams each day. To this point, I seem to have suffered no toxic effects, but must point out that I take the vitamin C in the crystalline form as a mixture of ascorbic acid and sodium ascorbate

††*And Now, in Summary. . .*

There is an old saying, "You pays your money and you takes your choice." Not very good English, but full of meaning. I have the greatest respect for the remarkable, indeed invaluable studies in nutrition reported by Dr. Jean Mayer. I also have the greatest respect for Nobel Laureate chemist Dr. Linus Pauling. Only time and considerable controlled experimentation on animals and man will provide the ultimate answers.

The health of your teeth is dependent upon the nutrients you provide in your daily diet. Follow the Revitalization Program and you will be offering your teeth, gums and the bone in which your teeth are set the best possible chance for long life and good health.

Add to this the daily local care with dental floss and so forth that you will learn from your dentist, and you have a good chance of going through the next hundred years with your own teeth, in good health.

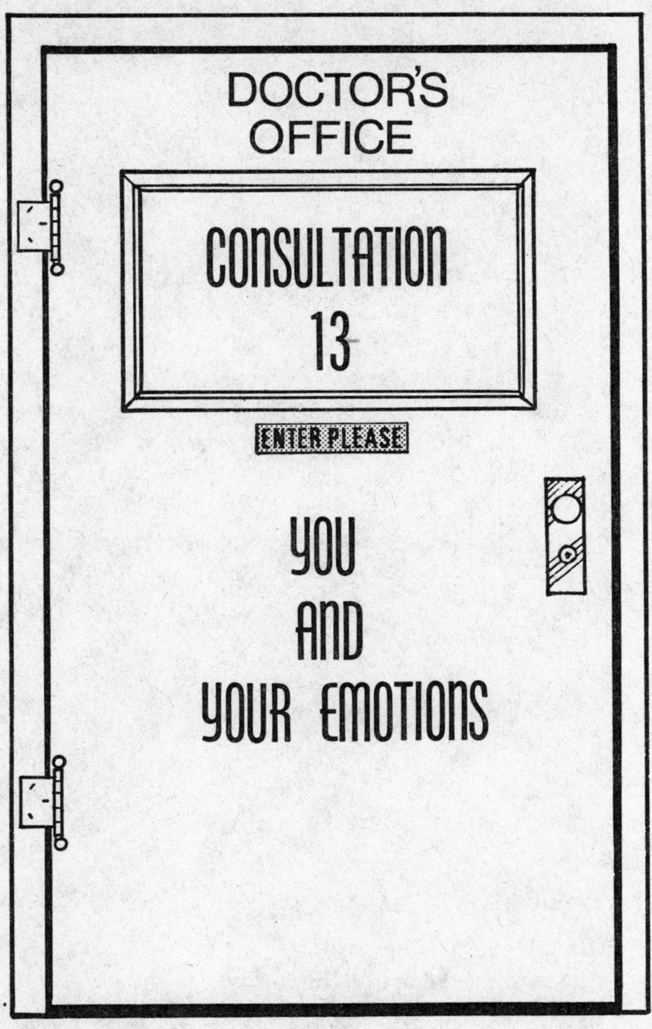

DOCTOR'S
OFFICE
CONSULTATION
13
ENTER PLEASE
YOU
AND
YOUR EMOTIONS

The Cantor Equation

There has been much confusion in the treatment of emotional disturbances of all types, including schizophrenia and other serious disorders of the mind-body. My concern in writing this consultation is that all mind-body problems lead to deterioration in the mind-body structures, with accompanying loss of vitality and premature loss of youth and strength. I do not propose to offer any basic treatment for mental disorders other than the total Revitalization Program. I am personally opposed to use of destructive approaches such as shock treatment—but then I am not a qualified psychiatrist.

Although I founded the Academy of Psychosomatic Medicine and am its President Emeritus, the proliferation of psychiatric offshoots for the treatment of mental and emotional disorders has been even greater than the rapid growth of splinter religions and leaves me somewhat dismayed. Indeed, both the growth and the underlying strength or lack of strength of such new ventures into spiritual spheres and psychiatric treatments seem to have much in common.

I will offer what I have called the Cantor Equation as a *tentative* structure upon which to develop the ultimate answer to the major factors in the search for basic answers for revitalization of the body-mind. This, of course, includes the *mental-emotional disturbances* under discussion, *as well as cancer.*

You will note that the Equation does not specify mental disease at any point. You may assume that it does, however, include such disturbances since the emotions may not only devitalize the body-mind, but can even kill the organism.

Basic Factors

Length of life, retention or revitalization of youth, and strength of the immune system, depend upon the following factors.

1. **The hypothalamus—thalamus—pituitary triad.**
2. **Stress, which mediates through this triad.**
3. **The release of thyrotropic hormone.**
4. **The effect on the thyroid-activation or thyroid-suppression mechanism.**
5. **The release of the (postulated) death hormone of the pituitary.**
6. **The degree of thymosin production (essential to adequate function of the immune system and its T-lymphocytes).***
7. **The level of T-lymphocyte pooling in the spleen.**
8. **Nutrient effect on all of the above.**

---

*The thymus is the master gland of the immune system.

9. **The RNA–DNA programming as it relates to cell life and its susceptibility to degeneration and/or regeneration via nutrition and hormones (oral, parenteral).**
10. **The stress-control mechanism available and activated.**

The Final Equation

Stress → Hypothalamus → Thalamus → Pituitary → Thymus → Spleen → RNA → DNA → Thyroid → All Endocrine Glands and Their Hormones → B- and T-Lymphocytes → Life/Death, Premature Aging or Revitalization and Rejuvenation.

Since this book and its consultations are intended for the layman, even more than for the physician-advisor of the devitalized patient, I will try to simplify the equation.

The controlling factors in determining how long we live, the state of our body-mind health and the goal of revitalization are listed from one to ten.

The brain segments at the base of the brain are the hypothalamus and the thalamus, which affect the all-powerful pituitary gland. All stress seems to be filtered through or originate in this triad.

Stress in small amounts is helpful in keeping us alive. In large amounts, it can overwhelm our internal defenses (all ten factors in the equation) and cause serious disease or death.

What you think, in other words, and how you react to stress can strengthen or kill, and the decision seems to be made in the hypothalamus-thalamus-pituitary area.

The pituitary is the body's master gland. It is even postulated that the pituitary has the power to retain or release a death hormone, but this hormone has not yet been isolated.

The thyroid gland may be activated or suppressed by the thyrotropic hormone. Again, the master pituitary gland seems to be in control, but only through the triad described above (factor one). Most of us need additional thyroid hormone to retain youth and energy as we grow "older," to revitalize our body-mind, but this can best be determined by your physician.

Thymosin (point six) is the "magic" hormone secreted by the thymus gland although there may be others. This gland lies behind the breast bone and shrinks with age. The T-lymphocytes, which fight cancer cells, must pass through the thymus. Thymosin is now under study as a potential cancer-fighting hormone. However, it is difficult to produce in pure form as a bovine source and is not yet available for human use except for experimental purposes. It is also very costly to produce.

The fighting T-lymphocytes are also pooled in the spleen (point seven), and if the level is low, the body has much less chance of containing and controlling cancer. As you can see, we are dealing with some of the basic elements of the immune system that determine how long you will live and perhaps how you will die.

There is little to be said about point nine. Our genetic structure is determined when the sperm meets the egg. But, it is subsequently weakened or strengthened by what you eat and what you think, as well as what you inhale. Eat the foods described in the Revitalization Program, live the life proposed therein and stay away from tobacco and poisoned-air environment. If you do these things, your inherited structure will have the best chance for survival and continued youth.

Point eight is what this book is all about. I do not need to repeat myself, but I suggest that you read and reread these consultations at least once a month for the next one hundred years.

Linus Pauling and Orthomolecular Medicine

Nobel Laureate in chemistry, Linus Pauling, has introduced the concept of orthomolecular medicine as "the preservation of good health and the treatment of disease by varying the concentrations in the human body of substances that are normally present in the body and are required for health." The vitamins play a major role in this concept, especially ascorbic acid (vitamin C).

This has led to the orthomolecular treatment of cancer in terminal cases with large daily doses of vitamin C, a reported increase in life expectancy of about four times the usual duration and improved quality of life during that time. This was described in the medical literature by Doctor Ewan Cameron and Doctor Linus Pauling in 1974.

A follower of the orthomolecular theory, Allan Cott, M.D., has offered a biochemical approach to the treatment of schizophrenia with orthomolecular substances. Nicotinic acid and nicotinamide have been in the forefront of the preparations used for the treatment of mental disease since 1952. The proponents of this theory of treatment believe that vitamins in large dosage may be the treatment of choice in mental disease. Since I have no personal experience with this form of therapy in the mentally and emotionally disturbed, I cannot comment further. But, as there must be a biochemical basis for schizophrenia, among other factors, it is important that careful study of these patients be made to better understand the pathology and direct the treatment.

As to revitalization of the body-mind, I can only confirm my belief that good nutrition, as defined in this series of consultations, is of basic importance to all of us.

Dr. Roger J. Williams, the discoverer of pantothenic acid, believes that a deficiency in niacinamide does exist in those with "mental disease" and that proper dosage with niacinamide may cure the problem. However, he bases this statement on the treatment of pellagra.

The Chemistry of Emotions

At a recent meeting (November, 1977) of approximately 4,000 or more neuroscientists (brain experts) almost 2,000 scientific papers were offered to describe the chemistry of the brain. It would appear that Sigmund Freud was quite right when he said that the answer to emotional problems was not to be found in psychoanalysis, but rather would be found in an understanding of the chemistry of the brain. The recent discoveries with regard to that chemistry show that ". . .we are beginning to see how chemistry actually causes us to behave as we do." That statement came from the outgoing president of the Society for Neuroscience, Floyd Bloom of the Salk Institute.

As I have stated in this book, there is a close relationship, apparently chemical in its control, between the hypothalamus and the pituitary, the master gland. The chemicals sent out by the hypothalamus apparently command the pituitary, which then sends out its own chemicals to the various organs under its control. There are more than 25 known neurotransmitters, and each neuron produces its own chemicals that send messages and orders to other neurons. One of the speakers at this important convention indicated that the patient with schizophrenia shows an increased amount of dopamine, a very important neurotransmitter in the brain.

It would also appear that our emotions, our moods, are determined by a group of chemicals produced by neurons in an "aminergic system."

It is obvious, therefore, that the brain must receive the best possible nutriton in order that its chemistry may function at optimal levels. That has been the theory underlying the concepts in this book. You need not understand the mechanism, the intricate details of the chemistry of the brain, but you certainly must understand that unless and until you provide optimal nutrition for the entire body, including the brain, the body will not function at its best levels. It may deteriorate, and it is entirely possible, in terms of the new understanding of the chemistry of the brain, that there may be a restructuring of some parts of the brain systems to replace areas which have been damaged by a lack of proper nutrients. This is further confirmation of the tremendous importance of proper nutrition as described in these consultations.

My Personal Opinion

I believe that patients with any form of body-mind deterioration deserve good nutrition, as defined in these consultations. They also deserve expert attention by specialists in the field of mental disorders, if that is their problem.

We are concerned in these consultations with body-mind revitalization, and this must always be a joint effort of the patient and the physician. I regret that I have no personal case histories to offer. However, this has not been my field of expertise, and I have always referred such problems to the appropriate specialist.

††*And Now, in Summary...*

Our goal is a healthy mind in a sound body. Since you are what you eat, what you think and what you inhale, follow the teachings in these consultations—the Revitalization Program—to develop your sound mind in a sound body.

Thought is not simply a product of the brain, and the emotions do not simply originate in the brain. Both thought and emotions, i.e., your mental health, are determined by the same factors that control your total body-mind health.

The Cantor Equation lists the major factors, and concludes that you require the entire Revitalization Program for healthy thinking and controlled emotional reactions.

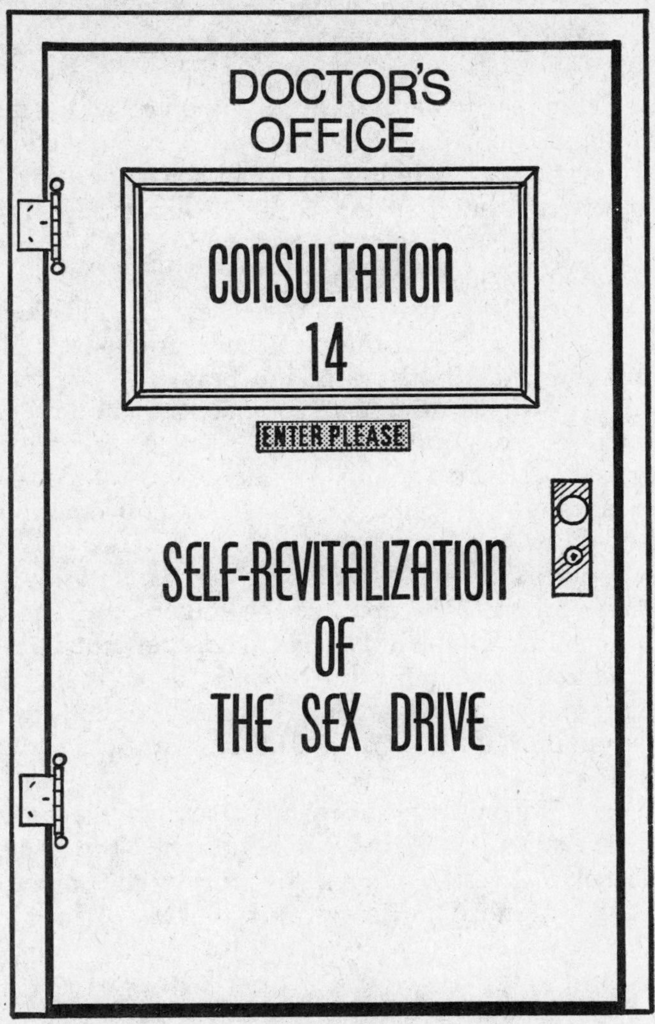

The General Approach

In this important consultation we will discuss the sex drive as it relates to depression of the function of the endocrine glands and, in many cases, how it relates to abuse of alcohol.

Self-revitalization is possible, even for those who seem to have abused alcohol to the point of "no return." Since the sex drive is seriously depressed in many alcoholics, we will discuss both endocrine and alcohol problems. We will offer a basic solution for sexual depression through our program of self-revitalization.

Let me begin by saying that without good general health, the sex drive wanes and sometimes disappears completely. Therefore, you must obviously follow the total self-revitalization program in order to strengthen every cell, every tissue and every organ in your body, including the endocrine glands and the sex glands and organs.

You have already learned about the importance of the endocrine glands and the fact that the pituitary is the master gland. If the pituitary gland at the base of the brain is not functioning properly, the sex drive will diminish. Since the pituitary gland is closely related to and monitored by the emotions, acting through the thalamus and hypothalamus at the base of the brain, the body-mind must be protected against stress and emotional disturbances of all kinds.

The best protection against such problems rests with the total Revitalization Program. The program, as you are now well aware, includes a great deal more than simply proper nutrition. It includes proper reprogramming of the mind as well and suitable exercises in conjunction with such reprogramming to increase the tone, the flexibility, the strength and the resistance of all the body tissues.

If you feel that you are losing your sex drive as you grow older, that is what is considered to be "normal." But it is not the optimal normal. It is really only the response of the "aging body" to the passage of time. This aging can be reversed, prevented or controlled.

Functional Menstrual Disorders

Menstruation is entirely normal. It is simply the natural body mechanism for discarding the womb lining if it is not to be used for a growing embryo. This means that the womb's lining is prepared for pregnancy each month, and if the pregnancy does not occur, the prepared lining is no longer necessary. So it simply detaches, and the menstrual flow represents this discarded tissue and blood. Obviously, there need be no fear, distress or anxiety about a normal process.

Menstrual periods will start at about 12 or 13 years of age and will continue to age 40 or 50. This is an inherited pattern. But, when the flow stops without warning you may become fearful that you are entering into an early menopause—aging prematurely. The condition is called amenorrhea, and it is simply the result of the emotions once again acting through the endocrine glands.

This can and often does occur at times of emotional shock, and you may expect that the menstrual cycle will resume once again when the stress is relieved. This has been seen constantly during times of war—in concentration camps, with bombings and with other types of stressful and inhumane forms of behavior. But, even the fear of pregnancy can stop the menstrual flow, especially if you are not married.

††*The Case of Miss A.*

Miss A. was eighteen years of age and unmarried, but living with her boyfriend. I knew both of these young people and realized that her problem was emotionally based when she stopped menstruating in consequence of the fear of pregnancy. All it required was a gentle discussion with both Miss A. and her young boyfriend to reestablish the menstrual cycle.

Any serious anxiety, fear, stress or shock can stop the menstrual cycle. With relief of the stress by reassurance, or by proper care from a psychologist or a psychiatrist, the hormone flow returns to normal and the menstrual periods resume.

We have exactly the opposite effect occurring when there is a swelling of the abdomen imitating a developing pregnancy in a woman who has a deep desire for pregnancy. This type of false pregnancy again reflects the remarkable influence of our desires, fears and emotions on the endocrine glands and on the functions of the entire body, especially the sex organs.

Later on, Miss A. developed another problem—painful menstruation. Again, this is a common functional disorder. Nevertheless, I referred her to a gynecologist, and he agreed that there was no physical cause. Here we find the self-revitalization program, especially the relaxation training and the positive self-affirmations, to be a great help.

I am pleased to tell you that Miss A. finally married (not the young man she was living with, but another) and had normal periods, three wonderful healthy children and is just now passing 60 years of age, but looking 40. She continued to follow the Revitalization Program in all its details and has thus prevented premature aging.

The Sex Hormones

Practically all women these days know that sex hormones (the estrogens) are available to maintain youthful tissues even after the time of the menopause, or to continue the flow at controlled intervals by the use of the proper hormone tablets. Most women taking these preparations also know that there are certain dangers. One of these dangers is the possibility of cancer of the breast and/or womb, apparently related to the use of the hormones. To my best knowledge, most of the women taking these preparations, so highly prize the continued or renewed youth resulting from the pill that they are willing to run the risk of cancer.

If they do decide to take this risk, and continue on "the pill," then they most certainly do need the best possible revitalization diet and the total program, in order to have the best possible chance of preventing or controlling the development of a malignancy. It is most important that women know that there is no loss of sexual desire with the "change of life." Indeed, it is usually precisely the opposite. Freedom from fear of pregnancy will often release repressed sexual drives. It may be hard at times for a man to satisfy the released female's sexual needs.

Even if no hormones are taken, you need not suddenly grow old during the change of life. Aging is a slow process, beginning at birth, and with proper nutrition, the aging process will become a slower, more controlled, less distressing factor in life. There need not be depressions, there need not be anxiety, there need only be a realization that the menopause is a normal process, and there must also be the appropriate provision of a very good diet as described in the Revitalization Program.

With reeducation, relaxation, self-suggestion and proper nutrients, the menopause need not be a serious problem. If you choose to take hormones, do so with a full understanding of the potential problems, and see your physician regularly so that you can have the appropriate studies and the necessary reassurance that all is well as you grow younger through your new lease on life, your new age of renewed youth.

What About the Male Menopause?

Impotence is a serious emotional-physical health-wrecker, but it need not be. I have found in my own practice, that through proper use of the male hormone in large doses by injection combined with the total Revitalization Program, male potency can be quickly and permanently restored. Indeed, I have seen patients become so much younger in appearance and sexual desire that they found it necessary to go beyond their wife, keeping one or two mistresses in order to satisfy their personal needs for sexual outlets. I could cite many cases, but the generalization that it does occur should suffice.

I will tell you about one patient, Mr. R., the very first that I treated in this fashion. Mr. R. had lost interest in life and was aging rapidly although he was only in his late forties; he had become impotent. With the loss of interest in life and in sex, he became a very unhappy, distressed individual. Fortunately, he had no financial problems at all, so he busied himself with his many important business ventures.

He developed serious headaches, wanted only to sleep at an early hour and even gave up television.

When he came to me for protruding, actively bleeding hemorrhoids, I removed them and he was very grateful. I casually mentioned the potential for a renewed sex life by injections, and he was interested but did not entirely believe it possible.

I told him that the hormones would work best only if he were in top physical condition, requiring that he change his diet, his way of life and his exercise program. He promised to follow the total Revitalization Program. With that promise, I began the use of male hormones (androgens), gradually increasing the dose until we found the appropriate level, so that he had no difficulty with erection at any time of the day or night. His desire for sex increased sharply, and in the past few years his capacity continues to increase so that now he not only satisfies his wife, but has three or four mistresses as well.

I have come to the conclusion that it is entirely possible to extend the life span in such cooperative patients to between 110 and 130. Naturally, we must all die. Most of us will come to the end of life in consequence of a heart attack or cancer. However, our best protection against both, assuming that we do not have a genetic predispostion, is the self-revitalization diet and program.

And finally, you may agree with George Bernard Shaw that it may be good to ultimately find freedom from the "tyranny of sex."

Alcohol-Pleasure or Poison?

It must indeed be obvious that, in small amounts, alcohol can relax and release you from tensions and some anxieties. Sexual activity may be enhanced or depressed by alcohol. This varies from person to person and depends upon individual tolerance. In large amounts, alcohol is a poison. Perhaps wine, in reasonable amount, with a meal, is the only time to take alcohol. You will note that I say "take" since alcohol is a potent "drug."

The cocktail party that ends in a sexual orgy, or in the death of a drunken driver after leaving the party, is an example of abuse of alcohol.

The question is not easily answered—pleasure or poison?. . .a pleasure in small quantity, and no danger to the sex drive. . .a poison in larger amounts, but how much is excessive? Again, each person is different.

You may say, "I can handle it." But, if you are hooked on alcohol, if you must have several cocktails before meals, or more often, instead of meals, then you may not be able to handle it.

Alcohol and the Revitalization Program

It is quite obvious that if you are a follower of the Revitalization Program and truly understand and follow its nutritional plan, you cannot possibly be or become an alcoholic. But, if you are already an alcoholic, you are now suffering from malnutrition. You need help from organizations such as Alcoholics Anonymous. You certainly need help in planning your diet. You desperately need to follow the advice in these consultations. I also recommend that you consult your physician and have him refer you to a competent psychologist or psychoanalyst.

††The Case of Jane L.

Jane L. lived and worked under constant stress. She was famous for her advertising agency and the originality she brought to her copy. However, like most executives under stress, her luncheons were mostly alcohol with relatively little good food as we understand "good" food. The luncheon cocktails and wines were followed by several drinks before dinner, and dinner was often a gala affair with several wines, followed by cordials and brandy.

Jane L. became an alcoholic. When she consulted me for vague intestinal symptoms, it was obvious that alcoholism was her major problem. I explained this to her, and advised that she consult with Alcoholics Anonymous as soon as possible. I told her that if she did not, she would soon enter into the irreversible stage of brain destruction, beyond which point little could be done. I also told her that her symptoms were primarily the result of malnutrition as well as the abuse of alcohol and placed her on the Revitalization Program.

My final words were those of encouragement, since she was very depressed during this consultation. "You are a very creative and successful person. You are attractive and young and have a long and happy life ahead. All you need to do is stop poisoning yourself. You are much too intelligent to commit suicide just to satisfy the custom of heavy drinking with your clients and your friends. Be as original in your life as you are in your business. Let the others do the ordinary and drink themselves into malnutrition and death. You do the original and say 'no' to the cocktails and the wine."

I am pleased to report that she followed my advice and now follows the Revitalization Program faithfully. She does drink, but limits herself to one cocktail before a business lunch. She had the strength to do this by herself, and did not join Alcoholics Anonymous as I had suggested.

Nutrition and Alcoholism

Although there have been claims that niacinamide and glutamine, as well as some other nutrients, are useful in the treatment of alcoholism, the evidence is not yet convincing. However, I have no objection to including these substances in the Revitalization Program if your physician so advises.

††*Your Prescriptions for Today...*

1. **It is possible to maintain continuity of youth throughout the menopause both for the male and the female.**
2. **A competent physician, the appropriate hormones, and the Revitalization Program make continuity of youth throughout the menopause possible.**
3. **If you are drinking too much alcohol and know it, there is hope for you. Consult with your family doctor right now, and if he agrees, join Alcoholics Anonymous. Your fellow sufferers who have kicked the habit will be your best friends and advisors.**
4. **If you can afford it, consult with a psychologist and/or a psychiatrist. Let your doctor guide you.**
5. **Start on the Revitalization Program right now. As an alcoholic, you are malnourished, and these consultations offer you the answer to that problem in starting you on the Revitalization Program.**

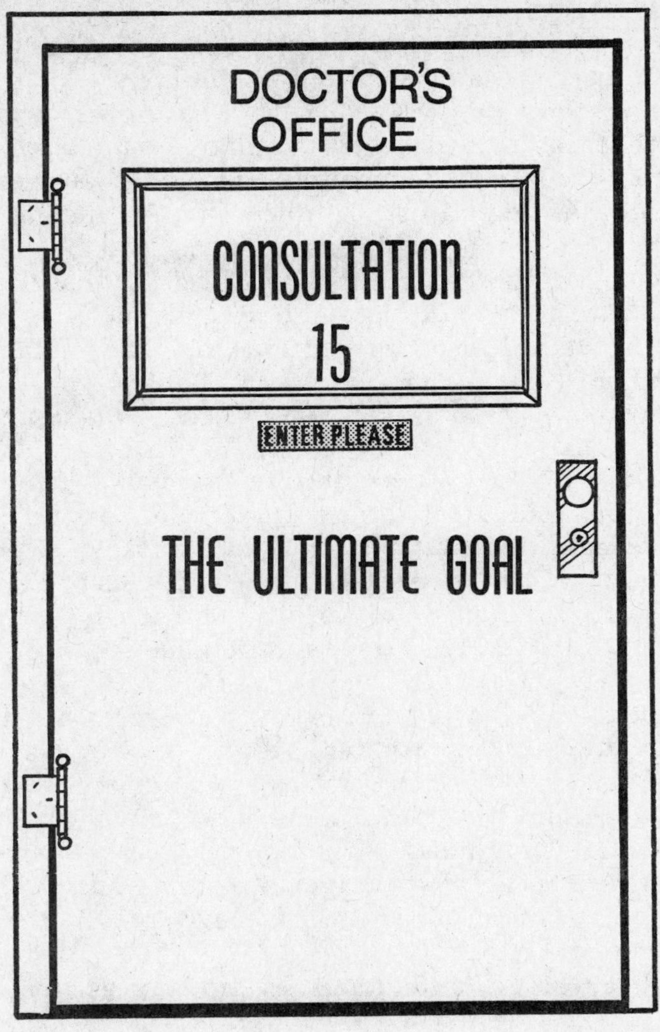

In this consultation, I shall simply tell you the case histories of twenty patients. The ultimate goal will be attained by you when you put the lessons learned into practice.

Only you can make yourself younger, restore health, prolong life and conquer death. Always remember that the power of healing is within yourself. Your immune system, your endocrine glands, every cell, every tissue and every organ of your body is under your control once you learn and practice the Revitalization Program.

I have consistently urged you to consult your family doctor, even a specialist or a surgeon. But, conquest of the ultimate goal of better health must begin with you. I have urged you to eat foods that will strengthen your body-mind—your total organism. These are natural foods, simply prepared, often raw, as in the Revitalization Cocktail. I have instructed you on the importance of the optimal levels of vitamins and minerals, and the dangers of going too far in the case of vitamins A and D. I have told you about the basic importance of the anti-oxidants such as vitamin C, vitamin E and selenium and where you will find them in natural, wholesome foods.

Always keep in mind that half-portions will lengthen your life and increase your vigor and health. Overloading your intestinal tract will overload all your body systems and reduce your resistance and your chance of prolonging youth and health.

I have instructed you in the dangers of tobacco, alcohol and caffeine beverages. If you are taking drugs (uppers and downers, or worse) you cannot possibly maintain good health. You will age prematurely and die before your genetic time-clock would have run out.

The lessons you will learn from the following twenty case histories and the lessons you have learned to this point will do nothing for you if you do not put them into practice. To read is easy, to act is sometimes difficult, but to continue the action each and every day is the most difficult. Nevertheless, I believe you can do it. And when you do, you will find yourself happier, healthier and younger, and you will live even beyond the age set on your genetic time-clock.

I wish you better health, longer life, and peace of mind for all time.

††*Case One—The Noted Psychiatrist*

We begin by looking at Dr. D., who consulted me well over thirty years ago. Dr. D. was and is a psychiatrist of repute.

His need was for lower bowel surgery, and the result was excellent. Fortunately, his condition was not malignant. Dr. D. was very fearful that it might have been malignant, since his sister and one brother had both died of cancer and both were in their early fifties at the time.

My surgery was performed in an operating room filled with soothing music and I operated with only local anesthesia so I could talk to my patient. We had a most interesting discussion on the merits of psychiatry, as well as reviewing its history and its failures.

When the operation was completed Dr. D., said, "I did not realize that you had begun."

I sent him home one hour after surgery, and he returned the next day for a dressing, feeling no pain. It was then that I told Dr. D. about the Revitalization Program, and he began to follow the precepts in earnest.

Dr. D. is now in his mid-eighties, very active in his practice, brilliant, alert and productive in every way.

He lives in a different state than I do, but we are in constant contact by mail and telephone. I often wonder if Dr. D. is my psychiatrist or if I am his, for I believe that our correspondence is so open and so interesting that it is keeping us both healthier and younger.

Is there a lesson to be learned from this case history? If so, you must find it for yourself. Only the understanding that comes from within yourself can restore your own health and youth.

††*Case Two—The Star*

This story relates to a young lady who is now quite famous as an actress. I will disguise her somewhat since we are using no clues to true identity in these consultations.

Lita C. consulted me for failing health and a loss of interest in living. She had never attempted suicide, but she had thought of it often. Indeed, Lita recounted to me vividly and dramatically, the many ways she had considered dying. I pointed out to Lita C. that what she was doing was the best possible therapy. She was living and reliving the problems and fears of her past in these fantasies.

Lita C. was happily married to a talented man and still carried on her acting career. She seemed to have no reason to want to die. Her general health was not as good as it might have been, since she could scarcely sleep through a night without waking at hourly intervals. We talked for about an hour during each visit, and Lita finally consented to try the Revitalization Program.

Whatever Lita did she did with great gusto. The importance of the healing factors within her own body was immediately evident to her, and she put her energies fully into preparing the Revitalization Cocktail in many personal variations, but always with the basic ingredients I had ordered. Lita C. loved the Buddha Dance, practiced the Buddha Walk, and was "enraptured" whenever she "conducted her own orchestra" to music in her own home. When she traveled she carried appropriate sound and cassette equipment with her so she could "conduct" in hotels or in the homes of those she visited. She soon had them doing the same.

Lita C. has lived a long life, and is still active. She wants to live another hundred years, and probably will! What lessons can you learn from her? There is a will to live and a will to die. Which do you choose?

††*Case Three—An Unhappy Millionaire*

The patient of my third case came to me as a young man who had already made a fortune in the stock market. He had started with little, sold short more than he bought long and soon had his first million. But the salt had lost its savor. He came to me in a serious depression. He had conquered the world too soon, and success had turned to ashes. He had no desire to marry. Indeed, he confided to me, he never would marry. It soon became evident that he had homosexual inclinations and was confused because he felt that this made him an "outcast." I reassured him, explaining that each of us is unique. His hormone balance was such that he was best suited for a life with another male rather than with someone of the opposite sex.

I told him that there was nothing innately wrong with this, since that was the way Nature or God had made him and homosexuality had been common since the beginning of time.

I did advise him to start on the Revitalization Program, since this would help him maintain and retain his youth and his strength, as well as prolong his life.

He was reassured, followed my advice and has lived successfully and happily ever since. He is now a well-known philanthropist and has put his money-earning capacity to good use.

Is there a lesson for you here? I do not know. For me there is the obvious realization that each of us must live in his own world. We are each unique. There is no ultimate reality. There is only your reality, my reality and so on, ad infinitum. There are as many realities as there are sentient beings in the world. You must live your own life in your own way to be happy.

††*Case Four—A Recovery from Stroke*

Death takes little bites, but a stroke is a large bite and can be terminal. Mrs. R. was only 50 years of age when she had a small hemorrhage in her brain, a "stroke" as it is commonly called.

Fortunately, she recovered without paralysis and decided that she had better change her way of living. She had been very much overweight, enjoyed rich desserts, drank alcohol heavily, partied late into the night and ignored her doctor's warnings. She knew that she had elevated blood pressure and was courting disaster but preferred to "live life to the hilt" while she could.

The stroke changed her attitude. She began taking the appropriate medications recommended by her family physician and slowed the pace of her life. When Mrs. R. consulted me as well, I advised the total Revitalization Program, especially the need to give up alcohol as completely as possible. She was now well motivated and had no trouble stopping her drinking. Although she had also chain-smoked cigarettes, lighting one from another, she gave it up, but she could not completely give up coffee.

I suggested that Mrs. R. taper off on caffeine in a gradual way, and after two months, she was down to only one cup after each meal.

The relaxation program was especially important for her, and she did this well. Indeed, she was in bed, ready for sleep, by five in the afternoon, practically each day.

Mrs. R. is now in her seventies, active in her own circles and seems both well and happy.

The lessons to be learned must be obvious in this case. The killers are alcohol, cigarettes, coffee and failure to follow her doctor's advice. The healers are the patient's own mind, the doctor's medications and the Revitalization Program.

More Information For You

I think that at this point I had better tell you more about high blood pressure and strokes. Loosely used, the word "stroke" means closure or rupture of a blood vessel in the brain. This is usually followed by paralysis in some part of the body, sometimes an entire side of the body. But there are smaller strokes caused by the rupture of tiny blood vessels or the blocking of those vessels from within by clotting of the blood where no paralysis results. But, there is brain damage, and brain cells do not regrow. The brain is the structure that represents the point of no return, because the brain cells you are born with are the only ones you will ever have. Many die each day, but since there are billions to start with, we can generally get by without even being aware of the loss. This is not so when there is a stroke.

Even when the loss is not severe enough to cause paralysis, there may be headache, diziness or insomnia, and you may tire easily. Your thinking may be less acute, and your personality can change, developing a tendency toward irritability and depression. Of course, you may not be aware of any of these changes, because they develop very gradually.

If you have not already done so, have your blood pressure checked at least once each year by your family doctor. If it is elevated, he will advise you on the proper treatment. You may need to lose weight. Or, perhaps, some prescription may be required. There are excellent medications that will assist you in lowering your blood pressure.

But, in my opinion, you must learn to relax, to roll with the punches and to change your dietary habits. The Revitalization Program will be the answer in many cases. Ask your doctor.

††*Case Five—A Severe Migraine*

Now I will tell you about Harry W., a young man with severe migraine. This form of headache is disabling. The structure and personality associated with migrane headaches may be inherited to some extent. The autonomic nervous system may be unstable (this part of our nervous sytem is not under voluntary control. It determines heart action and intestinal motion as well as most other internal functions).

Harry W. had severe nausea and vomiting with his headaches, sometimes heard ringing or saw bright or flashing lights. This is known as an "aura." When the headache began, he knew that he better get into a quiet room and avoid all contact with anyone. Harry could not stand noise or any other disturbance.

He needed good medical advice, and consulted a neurologist.

Even though Harry followed all instructions carefully, his attacks continued, although not as severely. Harry then consulted a psychiatrist, but he did not stay with the psychiatrist for long. A psychologist came next, and Harry stayed with her for a much longer time and did improve. His migraine attacks came less frequently.

Harry was on relaxant drugs, but he needed to learn more about how to relax. He came to my attention in relation to an intestinal problem, which I found was due to his anxiety state and was not organic. I suggested that he try biofeedback methods, or, if he preferred, simply put his feet in a pail of hot water as soon as he felt a migraine attack coming on. He chose the latter, and it helped "enormously." Harry A. then became most amenable to beginning the Revitalization Program in its entirety.

I urged him to continue with the psychologist since she was helping him understand his personality problems, in this case, his emotional immaturity.

††*Case Six—A Worried Lady*

Now, for a simple but very distressing type of problem. My patient, Mrs. V., was troubled by wrinkles. With aging, the skin usually loses some of its elasticity and wrinkles appear. What we do not usually realize is that the wrinkles we worry most about, those on the face, are the result of our own failure to relax the muscles of the face.

The muscles you must be particularly careful about are those around the eyes and the mouth, and those of the forehead. When you frown, purse your lips or squint your eyes, you are producing your own wrinkles, and they may become permanent. Here we must consider the importance of prevention. Of course, if you are on a proper diet, your skin will be more supple and less apt to wrinkle. The nutrients in the program described throughout these consultations are most important for good skin health. Vitamin C is essential for the production of healthy connective tissue, and when this connective tissue becomes sparse or hardened, the wrinkles are there to stay.

Mrs. V. was only in her early fifties but she looked seventy. She was not slim, she was emaciated. Diet to her meant not eating at all, and she lived on one small meal a day in order to "stay young." The effect was just the opposite. She had aged prematurely. I advised Mrs. V. on the importance of learning how to relax the muscles of her face, and told her about the total Revitalization Program. She was an apt pupil, and within eighteen months she looked, felt and behaved as if she were once again back in the early fifties. No salves, lotions or pills were prescribed, but she did use all types. I doubt that they do either harm or permanent good.

††*Case Seven—The Anxious Heart Patient*

Bob J. was first seen in my office almost 35 years ago, at which time he was 31 years old. His complaint was of palpitation of the heart. This meant that he was aware of the heart beating as a pounding in his chest. With this, Bob J. also had some shortness of breath, fatigued easily and had occasional chest pain. I suggested that his first stop should have been to a cardiologist, and Bob J. said that he had already seen several and none of them had found anything "wrong" with his heart. I telephoned one of the cardiologists he had consulted and was told that the patient had no evidence of organic disease and was simply suffering from fear and anxiety.

I tried to reassure the young man that his condition was sometimes called "the anxious heart" or the "effort syndrome," and that it did not represent any threat to life. Indeed, if he learned to relax and would follow my general instructions on diet, his symptoms would probably disappear over a period of time.

Bob J. asked me, "How much time? I could only respond, "That depends on you."

He began the Revitalization Program, but interrupted this false start several times. I did not see him again until three years had passed. By that time, he was one of the most relaxed persons I had ever seen. He had simply come to thank me and tell me that he was now entirely free from symptoms. Bob had married since I had last seen him, and was most fortunate to have found a young psychologist who truly loved, understood and guided him into following the total Revitalization Program.

He probably owed at least as much to his wife as he did to me, and I told him so.

The lessons to be learned are obvious. See a competent specialist, follow his advice and if not contraindicated, begin and stay with the Revitalization Program.

††*Case Eight—Another Heart Problem*

I call this condition the "tobacco heart syndrome." It also occurs in even more severe form when the patient both smokes and drinks caffeine to excess.

What constitutes "excess?", I personally believe that you should not smoke at all. If you take only one cup of coffee after meals, you are probably safe. Beyond that level, you are tempting fate.

John R. tempted fate. A successful broker, he smoked three packs of cigarettes each day and sometimes more. He drank "more coffee than I can count," day after day. The combination caused severe spasm of his coronary arteries, the blood vessels that bring blood to the heart muscle.

I told John R. that the cards were stacked against him, and he was doing the stacking. He had lost a sister from a "heart attack" at 41 years of age. He would be next if he continued to attack his heart with nicotine and caffeine. His general diet was not good. He was 31 pounds overweight, and he was beset with constant anxiety. John had consulted a cardiologist and was told that he had to lose weight, and should stop smoking cigarettes and drinking caffeine. But, since he was a stock broker and was on the telephone all day long, he found it difficult to break the habit.

His choice seemed simple. Stop or die. He made a valiant effort, gained and lost ground repeatedly over a period of the first year and a half, and then really mastered his emotions and remained with the Revitalization Program. John R. is now a very successful broker in retirement.

††*Case Nine—A "Problem Child"*

You now understand that your emotions may cause serious disorders in all parts of your body. The intestinal tract is particularly prone to such disturbances.

You may develop what I have called the "anxious colon," or the "anxious stomach."

Molly R., 34 years of age and a "fine wife," according to her husband, was an extreme perfectionist. Not a speck of dust in Molly's house! She even cut the grass, trimmed the bushes, did the painting where needed, and tried desperately to become the model housewife and a superb cook. Her husband appreciated her but looked elsewhere for companionship and sex, because Molly was too tired when evening came.

When Molly came to me as a patient, her symptoms were an overactive bowel and mucous in loose and frequent stools. She was convinced that she had cancer. Careful and complete examination, including X-ray studies of the entire gastro-intestinal system and an examination of the lower bowel with a sigmoidoscope (colonoscopy had not yet been invented), showed no organic disease.

My patient needed considerable reassurance, and I took a full hour to review all the studies and to assure Molly that she did not have an organic problem. What she did have was an emotional problem—a need to keep an absolutely clean, orderly and beautiful house. Indeed, it had become an obsession. I pointed this out to her and advised her to spend less time on the house and more time with her husband. I also urged the beauty parlor since Molly R. was aging somewhat more than she should, and had become thirty pounds overweight. Finally, I introduced her to the Revitalization Program as the best and shortest route to renewed youth, a slimmer, healthier figure and a new interest in life.

What lessons can we learn from this problem child? First, set a limit to your desires, even the desire to be a perfect mate. Second, remember that perfection may be an interesting goal, but it is not really possible for most of us. Third, a tired husband prefers a relaxed, fresh and attractive wife when he returns from the office or plant at the end of the day.

††*Case Ten—The Truck Driver*

Brad M. presented a more serious bowel problem, ulcerative colitis. In this type of case, the patient passes blood and mucous with the loose bowel movements. I first examined Brad M., a truck driver, over twenty years ago. He was a youngster of only 25, but I found extensive ulcerations throughout the lower bowel and much of the entire colon. Here we have a disease of unknown cause, and we must use every possible approach to attempt control of the symptoms and the ulcerations, as well as the weight loss and premature aging that always occur. There are medications to be prescribed, and the patient must be watched closely over a period of months or years, perhaps for a lifetime.

An emotional stress situation may precipitate this condition.

In the case of Brad M., it was the desertion of his wife, divorce and living alone for the rest of his life by his own choice, eating only the type of roadside food and drink most available to long distance truck drivers. I discussed with Brad the need for better food and supplementary vitamins and minerals, but he found it difficult to follow the recommendations. Finally, he gave up his job and took courses in plumbing. This was Brad's best move. He now has a large plumbing concern with many men working for him.

The pace of Brad's life is still active but does not contain the pressures and the irregularities of truck driving. He has settled down with a housekeeper who sees to it that he follows the Revitalization Program, and he has brought his colitis under control. There is no known "cure" for this disease, but control is often possible. In many cases, a psychiatrist or psychologist is needed to resolve underlying emotional stress problems. This patient did not need such care.

††*Case Eleven—The Difficult Doctor*

Dr. McC. was forty years old when he consulted me. He was also a victim of recurring bouts of ulcerative colitis. He lived the usual stressful life of a physician and added to this the stress of trying to become a championship-level golf player. Dr. McC. carried this to the extreme of carting a roll of toilet paper with him in his golf bag, playing even during times of bowel overactivity. He lived for golf. I think that it almost meant more to Dr. McC. than the practice of medicine.

But, he was a good patient and followed instructions to the letter. This is most unusual for doctors, who always second guess their personal physicians and rarely follow instructions. This patient, however, did exactly as he was told, took his medications regularly, and within six months, the diarrhea was under control and the bleeding had stopped.

Best of all, Dr. McC. finally realized that his goal of championship golf was an idle dream, merely a self-delusion. He became more relaxed and at ease, and he seemed younger. The Revitalization Program was, of course, tailored to his special needs, as it is in all such cases.

The lessons Dr. McC. learned were that, "although perfection is no trifle, trifles make perfection." The concept did not fit into his life pattern as a physician and a golfer, but he learned to strive for perfection in medicine and play golf as a hobby only. He learned to limit his desires.

You, too, must learn to set a limit to your desires.

††*Case Twelve—Ted L's Problem*

Constipation is a common, sometimes anxiety-causing problem. Almost everyone is constipated at one time or another. Ted L. was very constipated. He moved his bowels only after taking an enema, usually a soap-suds enema, as often as every three days. By that time, he had a full bowel of hard stool. My examination of this 33-year-old man showed no serious problem in the bowel. Ted L. had hemorrhoids, but they only needed injection treatment and no surgery.

His mother had given him a laxative every night of his life. When he left home and decided to give up the laxative habit, he became seriously constipated. It was the bleeding after the enema that bothered him even more than the constipation. Hemorrhoids (dilated varicose veins from straining at stool) were the source of the bleeding, and the injection treatment quickly controlled that problem.

I placed him on the Revitalization Program and suggested that he take three heaping tablespoonfuls of bran each morning in his breakfast cocktail. Within three months Ted L. was having regular daily bowel movements, completely emptying his lower bowel of stool each time. This bowel movement immediately followed arising in the morning.

Your lesson for today is obvious. For regular, easy bowel movements (assuming you have no organic problem) the proper diet will be your best bet. I hope you like fresh fruits and vegetables in addition to sunflower seeds and the all-important bran. All are important in developing a regular bowel habit.

††*Case Thirteen—Jane T's Pregnancy and Related Problems*

You might want to learn more about hemorrhoids. They are simply varicose veins in the rectum. Almost everyone develops them with the passage of time, especially if they are constipated. Merely assuming the erect position, as man does, is enough to produce a gravity effect in the lower bowel, and can produce hemorrhoids. Abuse of the laxative habit and poor eating patterns add to the problem for most of us. With straining at stool, constipation, or even diarrhea, the vein walls in the lower rectum are put under stress and weaken.

They may protrude with bowel movement, and then you have a double problem. External hemorrhoids may also develop when the veins around the outlet of the rectum weaken and dilate. It seems hard to believe, but practically all of us develop such weak vein walls and hemorrhoids, even in our early teens. Later in life, women have to contend with the pregnancy-constipation-hemorrhoid problem.

Jane T. was such a patient. She was pregnant, within a month of her delivery date and had bleeding hemorrhoids. Her obstetrician referred her to me for advice. Jane was anxious but not in pain.

I advised that she simply add the Revitalization Cocktail to her daily meal, with the permission of her obstetrician, of course. Beyond that, I urged Jane to wait until after the baby arrived to give the dilated veins a chance to restore themselves. If they did not, there would be time enough to consider surgery or injection treatment.

Jane T. followed my advice, had almost instantaneous improvement in her bowel movements after being on the bran routine for only three days and needed only injection treatment for the residual hemorrhoids after her baby girl was born.

††Case Fourteen—Excess Weight

Obesity is a major problem for both sexes at almost all ages. How do we escape the self-imposed fortress of fat? Elena O. presented herself to me simply for the purpose of losing excess weight. She was 50 years of age and looked 65. Grossly overweight, heavily made-up with cosmetics that simply emphasized her deep wrinkles—especially around the mouth, eyes and forehead—with the beginning of a dowager's hump, Elena truly needed help.

She said, "I have heard that you can make me younger. I responded, "Only you can make yourself look younger. All I can do is tell you how. But, more important than simply looking younger is to actually become younger. That can only be done over a long period of time, and only if you are willing to make a radical change in your way of eating and thinking and living."

Elena O. told me that she had been referred, not by her family doctor, but by a former patient and neighbor of hers who had seemed to "grow younger right before my eyes." I asked the name of the patient and immediately recalled a truly cooperative woman who had indeed shed many pounds and years to revitalize, and truly rejuvenate her entire body. Not having seen her in 12 years, I inquired as to her well-being. "She lost her husband in an airplane crash and has since remarried, a man years younger than she is, who looks 20 years older than his new wife." I realized that Elena was well informed and well motivated, so I started her on the total Revitalization Program.

Elena O. did exactly as ordered and has, in turn, restored new youth and vitality to her entire body-mind.

Your lesson for today is simply stated. You must be well motivated to stay on course if you are to revitalize yourself. The program described in these consultations is for a permanent life pattern of eating, drinking, thinking and, insofar as you can affect it, controlling your environment. I want to take a few moments to tell you more about environmental control.

††*Case Fifteen—Ask and you Shall Be Answered—Knock and it Shall Be Opened Unto You*

An apt Biblical quote. When you dine in a restaurant, do not hesitate to ask your smoking neighbors to please refrain from smoking. Tell them that you have cancer of the lung and would appreciate it if they did not smoke. This little white lie may save their lives as well as prolong yours. For your daily walks, if the air in your area is "unsatisfactory" as they say in New York City, do your walking indoors in an air-conditioned environment. At least some of the noxious elements in the air will have been filtered out. Be sure that you have fresh filters in your conditioner by checking the filters frequently.

When you have guests, serve drinks if you so desire, but do not try to keep pace yourself if your friends are heavy drinkers. Drink bottled mineral water (hard water), and if you must appear to be drinking alcohol, tell a little white, life-saving lie—"I drink only Vodka and water."

Ask for decaffeinated coffee in restaurants and in other people's homes if you are a guest. Everybody has it these days. Most people drink it themselves. You are not alone.

So much for the external environment.

Now for the internal environment. This calls for the Buddha Walk and the Buddha Dance combined with the repetition of "Younger and Younger, Healthier and Healthier," and so on, as you walk or dance. Do the same before entering into sleep. The Total Program is your best bet for renewed vitality and youth.

††*Case Sixteen—Suzy G.*

When treating the obese patient, it is important to take into account the patient's general condition. Often, there is a deficiency in thyroid hormone. This must be determined by the appropriate tests. Or, there may be a serious underlying stress problem. This may require the assistance of a capable psychologist or psychiatrist.

The lazy thyroid can occur at any age, but in my cases, the average has been well over 40. If the thyroid is not producing, you will gain weight no matter how careful you are with your diet—even if you are not overeating. Suzy G. had a lazy thyroid and became very heavy despite all her efforts to reduce.

With proper dosage of the thyroid hormone in pill form and with the Revitalization Program diet, Suzy became young again at 21 years of age. The loss of over 50 pounds made the difference between the older, former Suzy and the new Suzy.

I must caution you on the dangers of amphetamines in the treatment of obesity. You can become hooked on such medications, and they are not necessary in any case.

If you are overweight, your lesson for today is that you must see your family physician and have the proper studies to determine why you are overweight. You may need help for your endocrine and/or for an over-anxious, over-stressed mind-body. Since excess fat leads to many problems of a serious nature such as diabetes, heart disease, hypertension and stroke, bone and joint problems including arthritis and perhaps even cancer, it is a serious problem and demands your best efforts to lose the excess weight.

††*Case Seventeen—A Girl on Drugs*

Now we will talk about immaturity and its relationship to obesity. Most of us are immature in many ways. The alcoholic is certainly immature in continuing with the bottle as an adult. The patient who overeats to satisfy an emotional need is immature. The person who smokes cigarettes or marijuana, knowing that these are both dangerous drugs, is immature. It is not easy to grow up, but when you realize that the number of young people who smoke cigarettes is growing at an alarming rate and that the number of women developing cancer of the lung is rapidly approaching the rate among male smokers, then it becomes obvious that we are practically programming immaturity, programming cancer deaths into our population.

Our government is at fault in subsidizing tobacco growers and setting greater value upon the tax revenue from the cigarette manufacturers than upon the dying public who pay these taxes. Our cigarette manufacturers are at fault in doing the same—Greed rules the world.

Mary F. was 33 and very much overweight. She was also unhappy since her love affair had not culminated in marriage. "I wasted twelve years of my life on that man," she told me. They had been living together, in modern style, without benefit of marriage.

Mary found solace in both alcohol and tobacco, and sometimes (more often than she told me) was smoking "pot." Her diet was chiefly of the fast food variety, hamburgers predominating.

Mary F. was immature in many ways, but no one ever achieves full maturity. There is always some degree of immaturity, and most of us are addicted to one thing or another. But the degree of immaturity is what counts. Too much immaturity can hasten deterioration of your body-mind, thereby hastening death.

I referred Mary to a capable female psychologist who probably saved her from suicide. She did more for Mary than I could have done by diet alone, but when she consented to follow the Revitalization pattern, the result was most impressive.

She became a slim, svelte, very attractive young girl, and was easily able to reduce her drinking habit to an occasional cocktail. Mary gave up cigarettes entirely. I would like to report that she married happily, but I do not know.

Today's lesson? Try to see yourself as others see you. Be honest with what you see in the mirror, then decide for yourself whether or not you need help.

If you do, seek it at once. Do not delay.

Face the facts if you are a compulsive eater. If you are following a family pattern, face that fact and stop. If you are on the bottle, stop and ask yourself if you have really regressed to your mother's breast and the baby bottle. Self-understanding is half the cure; the other half is the Revitalization Program.

††*Case Eighteen—Amphetamine Danger*

Now, a further word of caution to stress the danger of drug treatment for obesity. The amphetamines or other comparable appetite-depressant drugs are central nervous system stimulants. They may make you jittery and cause elevated blood pressure in addition to getting you hooked if you like the feeling of nervous system stimulation.

Whatever weight you may lose when you are taking such drugs, you will probably regain rapidly when you stop. The problem is that you have never come near the reasons why you were overeating. Without finding the causes you cannot "cure" the problem. Obesity is a symptom as well as a disease.

John B., at age 45, is representative of the worst that can happen when hooked on amphetamines. John now visits a physician who supplies him with the large amount he requires to feed his habit—at a price. He refuses to stop since he is enjoying his "high" and thinks he cannot live without it. He is truly "hooked" on this drug just as the narcotics addict is "hooked" on narcotics. He refused to listen to his family physician, refused to even try to understand what I was telling him and continued on his regular round of amphetamines with the response, "I feel fine: why stop!"

There is no arguing with an addict.

††*Case Nineteen—Inability to Sleep*

Insomnia is a frequent and serious problem and may well be a major factor in premature aging. Jerry Q. suffered from insomnia, and could rarely fall asleep until at least six hours after going to bed. He then developed the habit of watching television until midnight before even trying to sleep. The result was that sleep did not come until three or four in the morning.

Jerry was, and still is, an active accountant, but the loss of sleep reduced his capacity to be alert during the day and he became heavily addicted to coffee. He took three cups after each meal and several in-between meals!

When I first met Jerry Q., he was in his early forties and looked tired, worn and haggard with good reason. To make matters worse, he had become further addicted to taking barbiturates and other types of sedatives and sleeping pills in an effort to cure his insomnia.

Obviously, sleep is essential. You may not require as much as others or you may require more. It is variable, and you may need as little as four hours of sleep to function well. Most of us need six to eight hours of sound sleep and some of us need a nap in the afternoon as well. Edison is said to have slept only four hours each day, but the fact is that he took naps during the day, hiding away in a small room.

If you feel well when you wake up and can perform well without drugs or caffeine in large amounts, then even as little as four hours may be all that you need. But, if you are not alert and fully alive during the day, you may need more sleep, even if you have already had eight hours in bed and asleep. Or, on the other hand, you may need a careful study by your physician to determine your basal metabolism—a thyroid function test and other tests.

I believe that a brief, untroubled sleep is better than a long, restless, troubled night of eight hours. Anxiety is a killer. Certainly, it will age you prematurely. Interrupted sleep, with difficulty in returning to sleep each time, is also insomnia and requires careful study and treatment.

Since your state of mind when you fall asleep is an important determining factor in how well you sleep, I urge that you follow the Revitalization Program instructions for self-suggestions, isometric exercises and so on before entering into sleep. The best time of the day to give yourself healing suggestions and to practice relaxation is just before sleep. Never miss this opportunity to restore your body-mind to better health.

Jerry W. was given a careful work-up and nothing organic was found to account for his problem. It was simply a matter of stress. He took his work seriously and was heavily burdened by a heavy overload of clients. I reassured him that he was not ill, but told him that he had to make some important changes in his life-style.

First, I suggested that Jerry take a partner into his office to reduce his workload. Then, I advised that he gradually reduce the amount of coffee he drank until he was down to one cup after each meal. When he reached that level, after six months, he was to become a drinker of decaffeinated coffee only. He did these things as I told him to. Meanwhile, I had trained Jerry in the total Revitalization Program, and he had become expert in instant relaxation.

He learned to relax the circular muscles around his eyes and mouth, to smooth his forehead and to quiet his mind, emptying it completely of the fears and the problems of the day. Next, Jerry repeated to himself, with long inervals in between, "Fully relaxed, at ease—sleep, sleep, sleep." With his body well relaxed and his mind emptied of the day's problems, the self-suggestions worked well and he was soon asleep. No more sleeping pills!

Jerry Q. became younger, more alert and alive than he had ever been. The lessons here are simple, and you can easily apply them to yourself. Avoid all drugs, if you can, unless prescribed by your physician. Avoid caffeine. Learn to relax both mind and body during the day, as well as at night. Reduce your work-load if you can. Set a limit to your desires, and you will find a way. Sleep well, and you will revitalize your body-mind and restore your youth.

††*Case Twenty—A Health-Wrecker*

Helen suffered from general anxiety, a very common, practically universal problem. That is why we see so many seekers after new ways of thinking and behaving, using the Oriental religions, Zen, Yoga and meditation in all forms. Unhappy and dissatisfied with life, often depressed—all suffer from what I have called a general anxiety syndrome. There are some answers to be found in the Oriental religions and practices. But the ultimate answer must come from within yourself. Indeed, that is the true goal of both Zen and Raja Yoga.

I have had hundreds of patients with this problem, and it is a basic health-wrecker. Anxiety is a form of stress. We all suffer from this at one time or another and some of us encounter it often or even most of the time.

Are we ever free from anxiety? I do not think so. Often, we carry the anxieties of our childhood and our middle years into our later years, constantly replaying them within our minds, consciously or unconsciously. This determines our attitude toward life and also determines our behavior.

The symptoms that result are often confused with various organic diseases. We experience the organ language of the brain, speaking through the medium of headaches, insomnia, obesity, nervousness, abnormal forms of behavior, vomiting, diarrhea and so forth. Anxiety may cause disturbances in the function of any organ or system of organs through overstimulation of the autonomic nervous system, the endocrines and the brain. See the Cantor Equation for the chain of command in Consultation 11.

Helen was 27 years of age when I first saw her as a patient. She had all the symptoms in the book and had been labeled a neurotic by her family physician. I found no evidence of organic disease and told her that she was suffering from general anxiety. I explained that this was not a disease, but that it could cause all the symptoms of many different disorders and had therefore confused her and her physician.

I suggested that she might benefit from consultation with a psychologist or psychiatrist, and she elected to see a female psychologist. I also advised her to change her way of living, her diet and her way of thinking. She was many pounds overweight, kept her hair and skin without regard for order or beauty, dressed as if she were fifty years old instead of twenty-seven and had generally let herself go.

She began the Revitalization Program and really gave it all her attention and energy. The result was astounding. Within six months, she had regained her self-respect, largely due to the psychologist's skill, but also in some measure to the new figure, the new attention to clothing and her new sense of self. She had indeed been revitalized.

You can do the same—the lessons are clear. Do not let general anxiety run you down and turn you off. Learn to understand yourself, and seek help if you cannot find the answers within yourself, your family, your past problems and your future fears. A good psychologist might be the answer for you.

If your general anxiety syndrome has caused disturbances in your body-mind functions, follow the advice of your physician, and if he approves, begin right now on the Revitalization Program.

††*A Few Words of Advice*

A good general, when outnumbered, may retreat. If you are in a state of general anxiety, then "run away"—take a vacation. You may even want to change your job, your place of living, even the person or people you are living with. But, before running away permanently, regroup your forces and make a stand. Take refuge in the Revitalization Program and return to the battle of life with new energy, new youth and new self-understanding.

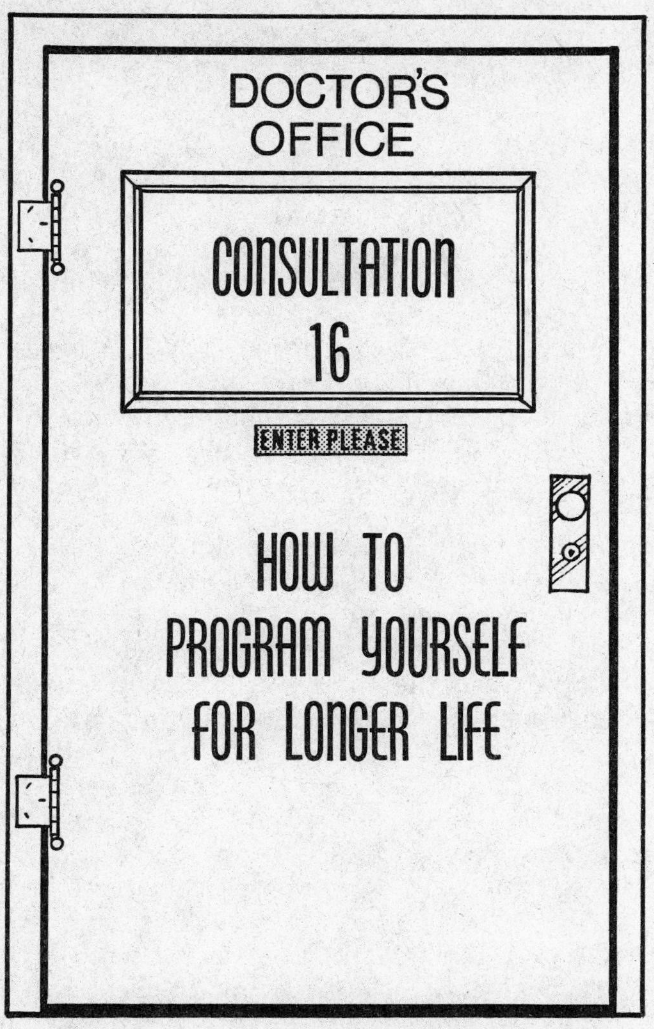

DOCTOR'S
OFFICE
CONSULTATION
16
ENTER PLEASE
HOW TO
PROGRAM YOURSELF
FOR LONGER LIFE

I have written extensively on longevity, and I would urge those of you who have not yet read my book, *Doctor Cantor's Longevity Diety* (Parker Publishing), to write to the publisher and obtain a copy so that you will have a basic understanding of my philosophy and practical approach to this question. During this consultation, I will give you some examples of my present thinking as they relate to the Revitalization Plan and longevity. However, it is impossible to provide—in a single consultation—all the material that you should know and apply in your daily life. You will find that data in the longevity diet book.

Key Word Control

During several of the previous consultations, I have taught you something about relaxation. I have told you how to relax in terms of relaxing during your daily life, at work, while sitting in a chair, while lying down and while preparing for sleep. All of these are important times and methods for relaxation.

I have instructed you on the importance of meditation during relaxation and whenever possible throughout the day. And I have also taught you how to use meditation and the various formulas of meditation in combination with relaxation. This is most important while sleeping. However, while practicing the relaxed Buddha Walk and the Buddha Dance, as described in our sixth consultation, you will simultaneously be meditating in the sense of using the special formulas to reprogram your mind with positive thoughts for better health and longer life. The combination of relaxation and the use of these formulas will aid you in deepening the relaxation, renewing energy and strengthening your entire body.

Now, I want to tell you about a rapid method to attain full relaxation called "key word control." When you have attained the capacity to relax completely by using any of the methods I have described above, you may begin the practice of key word control. The key word that you will use with be *Embee.* This is not a word that you will find in the dictionary, nor is it a word that you are apt to hear in daily life. It is a word that will be personally used by you to develop immediate relaxation at any time that you wish.

The origin of the word is the sound of the letters, M-B. This stands for mind-body, as you already know. Ours is a mind-body approach to revitalization of your entire body-mind. The sound of Embee is very important. It is a relaxing sound—one that you can repeat over and over and will find soothing to the mind and the body. Try it now, saying it slowly and repeating, silently or aloud—Embee. . .Embee. . .Embee.

This word, repeated slowly, represents to you in the future

and for all time, the entire set of instructions that you would ordinarily give your body to relax when you instruct the muscles of the feet, legs, abdomen, chest, arms, neck and head, one at a time, as previously described. This single word—Embee—will represent the entire set of instructions. This will now be your key word, and this key word will control the extent of relaxation and make it immediate, from head to toe.

First, of course, you must learn to relax in the fashions I have described in our previous consultations. When you have attained that degree of relaxation, working from muscle to muscle and from one part of the body to another, you may at that time substitute the key word to represent the entire process, and there will be instant and total relaxation. Now, you will find that as you continue to repeat the word, the relaxation will deepen. If you have difficulty sleeping, you will relax instantly, and fall asleep within seconds or minutes after beginning the constant repetition of the key word—Embee. You may use this word for total relaxation without going to sleep at any time you wish during the day. I would now like to tell about a very important executive who retained his position and revitalized his body and total energy capacity for work through the use of key word control.

††*How a Top Executive Stayed at the Top*

Lewis D. is a major executive in one of the largest corporations in America, based in the New York area. The stress of his work is enormous, his responsibility is international and his deals involve millions of dollars. Lewis D. is a man who has tried to keep in top physical condition by playing golf and tennis regularly. However, he combined his golf and tennis, as he did almost everything else, with business. The combination obviously kept him tense and under stress rather than relaxed and at ease. The exercise was good, but the stress counteracted it and resulted in loss of energy rather than in gain. Stressful exercise is harmful; it is self-destructive.

That is why I advise all my patients who play tennis or golf to play for fun; never play for money and never play for glory. This is one instance in which you can win the game and lose your life. If you play tennis, and otherwise lead a stressful life, I would suggest that you play only doubles. If you play golf, do not play to win; play for the exercise. Stress is a killer. The drive to be the best, to have the most, to achieve greatness, is the drive that calls upon your entire mind-body to expend energy. Most of us do not replace the energy lost, and the very process of energy loss simultaneously causes loss of vitality, often of the structure of important cells, tissues and organs.

Lewis D. first came to me because of an overactive colon that was so distressing to him that he had to carry a roll of toilet paper with him while playing golf. This became intolerable, so he came in for consultation about his overactive bowel. Careful examination by X-ray and otherwise showed no organic disease, but Lewis D. suffered from a very spastic bowel and an obviously very heavily stressed mind/body. I told this fine, fifty-four year old man, that he was on a path of self-destruction, a form of suicide. I asked him how much money he would take to commit suicide.

He looked at me as if I were mad. I pointed out to him that Howard Hughes had decided he had to have a billion or more and had withdrawn into the shell of a hermit and the mind-body of a very rapidly aging, depressed, paranoid individual in order to pay for his great fortune. The price he had set for which he would literally commit suicide, in my opinion, was one billion or more dollars. I pointed out that we are all of us committing suicide in one way or another, and the price may be glory, the Presidency of the United States or the accumulation of a vast amount of money. In the case of Lewis D., perhaps it was a combination of money and power. Whatever the motivation, it was self-destructive and therefore suicidal.

I told Lewis D. that his colon was simply responding to the stress that he had elected in driving so hard to attain and retain the top position in his organization. I complimented him on his attainment, but at the same time advised him that he was destroying his own life in order to achieve that position and remain at that level. However, it was only necessary to change his attitude, his way of thinking and his nutrition in order to revitalize his body and restore his capacity for work and self-fulfillment. I told him about the Revitalization Cocktail and the Revitalization Program, and I advised him on the matter of relaxation and the importance of reprogramming his mind-body in every way. His reaction was, "I will take it under consideration." It seemed to me that he would not return for further care and would most likely go his own way until death.

I was wrong, and six months later, Lewis D. came to see me. He was a man of action, and he had put my program into effect. He was now much more relaxed, and his colon, both on X-ray and in terms of daily activity, was no longer spastic. He had excellent bowel movements in the morning only, and had no diarrhea during the day. He had learned to play golf and tennis, "for fun, for the pleasure of it," and not to win. He had learned to modify his goals, which was, "easy for me, since I am already at the top." Lewis D. no longer, however, wanted to have "all the money in the world, or all the glory." This top executive revitalized his body, reprogrammed his mind and was on his way toward better health, renewed energy, revitalization of the body-mind and longer life.

Pituitary Concentration

The pituitary gland is the master gland of the body. It lies at the base of the brain, protected by a boney cradle called the sella turcica. The pituitary gland secretes a number of hormones, six of which can be clearly described and defined. The growth hormone determines how tall or short you will be. A hormone called "adrena-corticotropin" stimulates secretion of the adrenal cortex in the adrenal glands, one of which lies on top of each kidney. The pituitary also secretes a thyroid-stimulating hormone called "thyrotropin." This hormone stimulates both the formation and the release of thyroid hormones from the thyroid gland, lying at the base of the neck. The pituitary also produces a follicle-stimulating hormone that causes the growth of the important follicles in the ovaries of the female and controls the estrogen (the female hormone). It also acts, in the male, to control the formation of sperm in the testicles. The luteinizing hormone, also secreted by the pituitary, is the one that initiates ovulation in the mature follicle in the female. Without such ovulation, the egg would not be released so that the sperm could meet it to initiate the development of a new human organism. In the male this same hormone stimulates the testicle to produce the male hormone (testosterone). The pituitary also produces prolactin, responsible for the secretion of milk by the breast.

This is not the complete story, but it should be enough to indicate to you that the pituitary gland is indeed the master gland,

and controls most of the major functions throughout the body by manipulating the subsidiary functions of the other hormone-secreting glands in the body. Now, what do I mean by pituitary concentration? I have been a student of Yoga, Zen and meditation of all types for the past fifty or more years. In consequence, I have learned to place myself into a state of deep relaxation, using one or more of the methods that I have already described for you during the course of these consultations. In that deep state of relaxation, I have been able to focus my attention on what is called the "third eye" in the literature of the East. The third eye, in my opinion, really anatomically refers to the pituitary gland, the master gland of the body. When my full attention, my total awareness, is concentrated on the region of the pituitary gland, I begin to hear, at the base of my brain, a peculiar high level but gentle whistling sound. I believe this reflects the circulation in the region of the pituitary gland.

When this occurs, my entire body-mind is in a state of almost suspended animation, ready to receive whatever command I may wish to order. It is again my personal belief that in this fashion I can issue commands to the master gland and, through that modality, control much of my body function. I should say my body-mind function. I can deepen the relaxation to an almost unbelievable extent, practically to the point of suspended animation or hibernation. I can produce instant dreamless sleep of whatever depth I choose. I can sufficiently energize my body in this fashion so that each minute of this type of deep relaxation (at the "hibernation" level) is equivalent to one hour of stage four or very deep sleep. Thus, eight minutes of such hibernation sleep is equivalent for me to eight hours of ordinary sleep. It is my opinion that anyone can do this with proper training, and that this training can come from within yourself. Indeed, it must because no one can do it for you.

Practice the relaxation techniques that I have been describing, as often as you can. Place yourself into a deep state of relaxation just before going to sleep, and issue the command to the "third eye" at the base of your brain that "each minute of deep relaxation will be the equivalent of one hour of stage 4 sleep." During stage 4 sleep there is no dreaming. It is the deepest level of sleep. It is the most relaxing and reenergizing level of sleep. Then, let yourself drift off into sleep.

You may prefer to try this at a time when a nap is possible, but only a short time is available for such a nap. A brief nap, as brief as eight minutes, will give you the equivalent relaxation, revitalization and energy of an ordinary eight-hour sleep. This will become possible for you if you have the capacity to relax completely, focus your attention at the base of your brain and issue your command to the master gland.

I am not saying that everyone *can* do this. I am only saying that if I can do it, there is no reason in the world why anyone should not be able to do the same. It is not magic, not occult, not mysterious. It is merely an excellent example of how the mind-body functions as a single unit. When you focus your mind to cause the contraction of your fingers to form a fist, you do not consider this to be mysterious or occult. Why should you consider it mysterious when you focus your mind on the pituitary gland at the base of your brain and command it to function as described? I must caution you that I did not learn to do this in a single day, in a month, or in a year. However, gradually, over the course of several years, this became not only my potential, but an act of reality. It can become the same for you.

For those who think that what I have described is "way out," I refer you to *Fortune* magazine of December, 1976, on page 152 describing "Future drugs that will be life savers." On page 154 they speak of the "Yin-Yang" theory in connection with alterations of the cellular mechanism of the human body. They state that "this dualism in biological control has inspired. . .a Yin-Yang hypothesis for such alterations, patterned on the ancient Chinese ideas that alternating light and darkness are the determinants of life." Does that sound, oriental, occult? Of course it does. But it is basic to life processes, and basic to the understanding of the important functions of all human cells.

This particular article dealt with the way the human body manufactures its own wonder drugs, especially one of the body's best defenses against infection by viruses. That internally produced wonder drug is called "interferon." Major drug companies are putting vast amounts of money into the study of these natural substances produced by hormones within the body to fight disease and restore health to the cell, the tissues and the organs under attack by infection or cancer.

One of the researchers mentioned in the article is Dr. Choh

Hao Li of the University of California's Medical Center in San Francisco. Over ten years ago, Dr. Li located a new hormone related to fat metabolism. This hormone, lipotropin, contains substances that act as the brain's "own morphine-like pain killers." Please remember that we are talking about the hormones in your body and in mine, and when I speak to you about your innate (but as yet uncontrolled) capacity to relax the body or stimulate it, I am speaking in purely scientific terms. This is neither occult nor mystic. It is something that you can indeed learn to do if you have the desire and are willing to follow my instructions.

††*How Andrew F. Learned to Stop Worrying*

I had known Andrew F. as a neighbor in our community for many years. He was in his early fifties and successful in his business of manufacturing umbrellas, but he was constantly unhappy and constantly worrying. He worried not only about the market for umbrellas, the competition from Japan and whether or not it would rain sufficiently during the coming year, but he worried about absolutely everything else in the world. He worried about the children dying of malnutrition in India, he worried about the children dying of leukemia in the Sloan-Kettering Memorial Hospital in New York. Andrew F. had come to the conclusion that everything man has ever done, is doing or will do, has been, is and will be totally worthless and meaningless.

I believed that Andrew was enjoying his worrying, but when he developed severe angina pectoris, combined with almost every possible type of gastrointestinal symptom, it became evident that he really had something to worry about. It was then that he spoke to me, informally, during a luncheon that he had arranged for the two of us. When I saw the type of food Andrew F. was accustomed to eating, the great speed with which he stuffed his mouth and swallowed the food, practically without chewing it, I knew that he did indeed have something to worry about.

He asked me if I thought I could help him with his various problems, especially the overactive bowel, the feeling of nausea and the desire to vomit after practically every meal. Since he had already visited many physicians and had undergone numerous complete studies, it was not necessary to repeat these procedures. He truly had severe angina pectoris, hypertension and all the stress-related problems that were taking their outlet through his intestinal tract. I told him that I would be willing to accept him as a patient only if he would in turn be willing to listen instead of talking constantly about the state of the world, the hopelessness of man and his activities.

I assured him that, in the first place, I completely agreed with him. Man is indeed the most destructive animal that ever lived. He is the only animal alive I know that kills for pleasure. All other animals kill only for food or in self-defense. Man is the only animal I know that accumulates bits and pieces of paper called money, bits and pieces of metal such as silver, gold and copper, with an insatiable desire to have more, and more and more. He is never satisfied while other animals are satisfied when they have sufficient food, clothing in the natural form of their fur coats or other outward skin protection and shelter.

I told him the most enlightened Zen Master had come to the conclusion, centuries ago, that the best way to live is with the understanding that "when I am hungry I eat—when I am tired I sleep." I asked my friend if he could, at this time or any future time, see himself setting a limit to his desires. I meant not only the desire to accumulate, but the desire to change and reform the entire world. I pointed out to him that it can't be done. Indeed, great civilizations had disappeared from the face of the earth during the course of the many centuries since man began to despoil this planet. Andrew F., too, would soon leave this world—and take his worries with him if he did not learn to stop them.

I pointed out to him that he was obviously enjoying his worrying, but at the same time subjecting himself to enormous stress. That stress was now showing itself in the various symptoms and serious disorders that had affected his gastrointestinal system and his cardiovascular system. Andrew agreed to follow my instructions, and I started him immediately on the complete Revitalization Program. It was obvious that he had to change his way of eating, his way of thinking and his way of living in a very radical fashion. I made it quite clear to him that his life was at stake.

From this point on he had nothing to worry about except survival. He had to learn to live, I pointed out to him, one day at a time. No one has more than one day at a time. It is certainly obvious that this could well be the last day for any one of us. It is better, however, to take the positive attitude and think that this is the first day of the rest of your life. "If you succeed in your survival program," I told him, "you will have many more years ahead of you to live and enjoy life—hopefully without the worrying. But if you cannot do this, you cannot expect to even survive let alone live a long life, unless you change your ways of thinking as well as your ways of living."

I taught him the Buddha Walk that very day. Within a week I had advanced him to the Buddha Dance. He was very adept at the practice of the meditation formulas, had quickly achieved the capacity to relax completely and was well on his way toward key word control of that relaxation. I am pleased to report that Andrew F., the chronic worrier, is now a confirmed optimist who lives one day at a time and expects to be here the following day. He is in his seventies and will probably outlive all of us. He had learned to stop worrying and start living.

The Master Gland and You

You have already learned a great deal about the nature of the pituitary gland at the base of the brain, its functions, and how you might achieve the capacity to control and direct those functions. You realize that the master gland determines practically everything that goes on in your body-mind through its innate capacity to form hormones that in turn act upon the other major endocrine glands of your body such as the thyroid gland, the adrenal gland and the ovaries and testicles. Now I ask you to take a giant leap forward in your thinking and try to understand the following concept.

You *are* every cell, every tissue, every organ, every part of your body. That should be obvious to you. That is what you truly *are.* You are, therefore, the pituitary gland. You *are* therefore,—obviously—in control of your entire endocrine system. It is you—your mind-body—acting on the pituitary gland and through the pituitary gland, that control all the major functions of your entire mind-body, all the functions of every cell, every tissue and every organ of your body. Stop now and try to internalize this important concept. *You are the master gland.*

Lie down now and relax. Attain the deepest relaxation you possibly can and repeat to yourself, "I am the master gland. I am the pituitary gland, lying in my protective boney structure, the sella turcica at the base of my brain. I am in total control of this mind-body." Do you truly understand this? Do you truly realize that you are indeed the pituitary gland, a master of your mind-body; master, insofar as that is possible for anyone, of your own destiny? When you do achieve this state of understanding, this degree of comprehension, you will be in control of all the functions of your mind-body.

Your next step is simply to provide your master gland and all the other cells, tissues and organs of your body with proper nutrients and the positive type of thinking that will make it possible for the master gland and its servants to function at an optimal level. That function will then take place in a mind-body that is healthier and healthier, happier and happier, younger and younger, every day in every way.

If you truly understand what I have just said—and this is perhaps the most important conclusion in this entire volume, in this entire set of consultations—you will control your own destiny insofar as that is physically and mentally possible.

More on the Master Gland

A recent article in the New York Times, written by Harold M. Schmeck, Jr., describes the role of the pituitary gland in producing substances similar in action to the opiates. I have already described this important finding, as reported in Fortune magazine in 1976. But Mr. Schmeck brings us up to date in a most interesting fashion. He reports that the new discovery "opened up a new realm of body chemistry offering clues to the nature of pain, pleasure, and perhaps such matters as epilepsy, drug addiction and mental illness."

The new morphine-like substances are called the "endorphins," translated as "the morphine within." There may even be a relationship to depression and schizophrenia, and if this is so, the possibilities for revitalization in such conditions are now extended far beyond our present forms of treatment. There is even the possibility, he reports, that the drug addict may be born with a "natural deficiency" of endorphin production. The reverse would be true for those who are relatively free from pain under conditions that would require pain-killers, even narcotics, for most of us.

We know that pain is primarily an emotional response, but

now we have a definite link with the pituitary gland and, no doubt, with the thalamus and hypothalamus at the base of the brain. I will not go into the many theories or the experimentation and study now going on in this important field. They are very complex and do not lend themselves to firm conclusions as yet.

At a recent meeting of approximately 4,000 or more neuroscientists (brain experts) almost 2,000 scientific papers were offered to describe the chemistry of the brain. It would appear that Sigmund Freud was quite right when he said that the answer to emotional problems was not to be found in psychoanalysis, but rather would be found in an understanding of the chemistry of the brain. The recent discoveries with regard to that chemistry show that". . .we are beginning to see how chemistry actually causes us to behave as we do." That statement came from the outgoing President of the Society for Neuroscience, Floyd Bloom of the Salk Institute.

As I have stated in this book, there is a close relationship, apparently chemical in its control, between the hypothalamus and the pituitary. The chemicals sent out by the hypothalamus apparently command the pituitary, which then sends out its own chemicals to the various organs under its control.

There are more than 25 known neurotransmitters, and each neuron produces its own chemicals that send messages and orders to other neurons. One of the speakers of this important convention indicated that the patient with schizophrenia shows an increased amount of *dopamine,* a very important neurotransmitter in the brain. It would also appear that our emotions and our moods are determined by a group of chemicals produced by neurons in an "aminergic system."

It is obvious, therefore, that the brain must receive the best possible nutrition in order for its chemistry to function at optimal levels. That has been the theory underlying the concepts in this book. You need not understand the mechanism or the intricate details of the chemistry of the brain, but you must certainly understand that unless and until you provide optimal nutrition for the entire body, including the brain, the body will not function at its best levels. It may deteriorate, and it is entirely possible in terms of the new understanding of the chemistry of the brain that there may be a restructuring of some parts of the brain systems to replace areas which have been damaged by a lack of proper nutrients.

This is further confirmation of the tremendous importance of proper nutrition as described in these consultations. But the conclusion we can draw is that if we can somehow learn to relate to and control the pituitary-thalamus-hypothalamus complex, we might very well be able to better control our emotions, stressful problems and, perhaps, even pain. That is our goal at the present time, and I have offered my own concepts as to how we might proceed.

You must learn how to relax, how to roll with the punches in countering stress, and how to relate to your pituitary gland by focusing your attention on its approximate location and ordering it to do your bidding.

If you succeed in doing this, you will have taken a giant step ahead in your search for longer life and better health.

The Effect of Redirection

Let us continue with our thinking in terms of the fact that you are the master gland. Indeed, you are every cell, every tissue, every organ of your body, and they, in turn, are the products of one factor you cannot control—the genetic factor—and other factors that are within your complete control. The nutrition you provide for these cells in terms of food for the body and food for the mind is one of these factors. Having understood this, you need only redirect your life patterns in terms of the food you provide your body and the food you provide your mind. I mean, of course, the total mind-body, the unity of mind and body that represents you.

The effect of such redirection will obviously be to improve the function of your mind-body. You will do it under your own control and under your own direction. You will do it of your own volition. You will do it with the understanding that *you* are now in control of your own destiny, insofar as that is possible in this amazing world of chance.

A few words about chance. It was chance that brought a particular sperm to a particular egg, resulting in you. It was chance that determined the type of tissue with which you were born and the total mind-body pattern. But think how wonderful even that was. You are representative of a chain of life that goes back to the beginning of time. An unbroken chain. If you have children, that chain of life will continue.

In sum, then, you are—barring chance—in total control of your destiny. You are the master gland. You are each cell, each tissue, each organ of your mind-body. If things are not going well, all you have to do is change the direction by providing proper food and proper thinking for your mind-body. Instruct your master gland—for you are that gland—as to exactly what you wish done. If the process of self-destruction has not advanced too far, you can revitalize your mind-body, restore new energy, new point and purpose to your life, restore at least some degree of new youth and very possibly ultimately achieve the one-hundred or more years of long, happy living that you are striving for.

††*How John L. Achieved Long Living Potential*

I have emphasized, throughout these consultations, the great importance of nutrition in reconstructing, revitalizing and reenergizing our defense mechanism in terms of the immune system. A Professor of Surgery at the University of Cincinnati Medical Center, J. Wesley Alexander, M.D., speaking at a Symposium in Boston, Massachusetts, reported that the clinician's most fruitful approach to correcting defects in defense is by way of nutritional supplementation. He pointed out that it has been documented that malnutrition not only impairs neutrophil function but reduces complement levels and activity. It also inhibits antibody synthesis and impairs T-cell function. The importance of this is great since most surgical patients become infected, not as a result of some defect in B-cell or T-cell mediated immunity, but rather because of a defect in monocytes and neutrophils. The increase of these cells by an antibody that acts as a specifier and by complement, functioning as an amplifier of that specification, is the underlying mechanism.

Do not be concerned by the technical nature of this report. The important statement is that your immune system is best improved, sustained and reenergized by nutritional supplementation. That is the message of these consultations.

John L. was suffering from malnutrition, not because he could not afford to eat, but because he did not take the time to eat. When he did take the time, it was at quick food restaurants—a hamburger, french fried potatoes, a soft drink. And, of course, he consumed large amounts of coffee. He felt that he was eating well, but his body knew otherwise. When John L. visited me, it was because he was constipated and experienced hard bowel movements which caused bleeding from the rectum. Careful examination showed no serious organic disease. I asked him about his diet, and the answer was very much what I had expected. I told him that he was suffering from malnutrition, and he said, "I thought that occurred only in countries like India." I corrected him by telling him that most people are suffering from poor nutrition and that his was very poor indeed. Although India suffered mostly from an inadequate supply of food for its tremendous population, the Americans suffered as well from a poor quality of food in great abundance.

I told John L. about the Revitalization Plan, the Revitalization Cocktail, and the M-B method of programming the mind and the body by providing proper food for thought and food for nutrition. All of these ideas were entirely new to him, and he accepted them eagerly and followed them faithfully. Within six months, John L. had recovered completely from his constipation, no longer showed any bleeding with bowel movements, had easy bowel movements regularly each morning and told me that he had never felt better. Since he was a young man, in his late twenties, he had achieved long living potential by a simple change in nutrition.

I am happy to report that John L. followed my instructions faithfully, and thirty years later was a very successful man in his chosen field as well as in his tremendous capacity for the enjoyment of both life and work. He had been completely revitalized, and was on his way toward "one-hundred-plus" years of long happy living.

Positive Thinking for Better Health

It has been wisely said, "Man is just about as happy as he makes up his mind to be." Try to take a positive attitude toward life. Certainly, life is a war between yourself and everyone else, sometimes yourself and your government, between yourself and your spouse, yourself and your employer and so on. In this war, you won't win all the battles, but you don't even need to try. Be content to win some and to enjoy all of them. It seems odd to advise you to enjoy the battles of life. But, since life is made up of compromise as well as struggle, learn to compromise and to retreat when necessary. Napoleon won many of his battles, but he knew when it was necessary to retreat, to withdraw and regroup his forces. You must also learn this important lesson. Practice looking at the bright side of everything. Smile as often as possible. Learn to laugh even when you fall down. Pick yourself up, dust yourself off and continue onward. Remember that you are what you think as well as what you eat. If you think happy thoughts, healthful thoughts, positive thoughts of success, revitalization, restoration of energy and health, you will assist your mind-body in achieving those objectives. Remember the important meditation, "Healthier and healthier, happier and happier, stronger and stronger, younger and younger." Reprogram your mind with these positive thoughts whenever you feel down. They will immediately give you a lift, and when your spirits rise, you will feel happier, younger and stronger, and your energy will indeed be renewed.

In terms of your health, although you are as old as your arteries, bring to the forefront the positive understanding that your arteries can be made young again. Your heart can be made stronger again. Your energies can be renewed, your immune system can be strengthened and you can become—in effect—younger, healthier, and happier. All of this can be accomplished by positive thinking and positive action in terms of revitalization.

Learn to give your full attention to the present moment. After all, this is the only moment you can truly live. You must live each moment to the full if you are to enjoy life. When you give your full attention to the taste of your food, your food will taste better and will give you more pleasure. When you give your full attention to whatever you see, hear, feel and touch, you will appreciate these sensations more than ever before.

When you learn to live and not simply exist, you will be in closer touch with the reality of life. You will see the world with a happier heart and a singing, joyous memory will remain. You must learn to count your blessings each moment of each day. The most important blessing of all is the fact that you are alive. You may not be entirely well, you may not have the energy you would like to have, but if you truly practice everything you have learned during these consultations, you will be well on your way toward a happier, healthier life. Remember that all you have to do is survive, to stay alive, and you will outlive your enemies and your troubles.

Try to make new friends every day, but don't forget to keep your old friendships by expressing your appreciation wherever possible. There is an old saying that "new friends are silver, but old friends are gold." Set a limit to your desires and keep your life simple. Think happy thoughts and let yourself be happy.

Remember that stress is the killer, but you can overcome stress by thinking happiness, good health, good fortune and healthier youth. Use the meditation formulas exactly as described and you will overcome all problems. Your subconscious mind will take over as soon as you have programmed it with the positive thoughts of new energy, new happiness, new youth and new life. The road to revitalization starts with a path that leads from the mind to the body, always remembering that the mind-body is a single unit. Positive thinking will give you better health.

††*How Ronald D. Prevented a Second Coronary*

Ronald D. experienced his first coronary occlusion at thirty-two years of age. He thought that he was in excellent physical condition because he jogged several miles each day. But it was during jogging that he had his first heart attack. Fortunately, he survived. His hospital stay in the intensive care unit was a difficult time for him. He could not understand what had happened since he was taking such good care of himself and exercising strenuously each day. He consulted me almost one year after this heart attack. He was depressed, confused and the effect of the stress was activating his colon to the point of almost constant frequent, loose bowel movements.

Nobody gave Ronald D. any instructions regarding diet. He was simply told to "take it easy", and to avoid stress, and was given the necessary medications to quiet his bowel. I discussed the problem with Ronald D. in terms of the Revitalization Plan. He was to exercise, but not by jogging. I recommended the Buddha Walk for him, and once he could do this without shortness of breath, I then recommended the Buddha Dance. However, the approach was to be a relaxed approach, in which he avoided stress at all times.

As for diet, naturally, the program was to be the one we have discussed all during these consultations. I told him that if he followed this plan carefully there was a good chance that he would revitalize his heart and arteries, and reestablish his past energy. But, he could not be impatient, and he had to practice the meditation formulas not only at the time of the Buddha Walk and the Buddha Dance, but always before going to sleep at night. The special formula for him was, "Healthier and healthier, every day in every way, healthier and healthier, younger and younger, stronger and stronger."

Ronald D. has never had a second coronary. He is now relaxed and is enjoying life—thirty-two years later.

Positive Action for Happier Living

Positive action requires a positive attitude toward life. It requires a positive attitude toward finding a solution for your immediate problems. It requires a positive attitude toward following the instructions throughout these consultations, especially to those relating to facing problems as they arise, seeking solutions and acting promptly. If you do this with regard to your health, you can expect revitalization of your mind-body. If you do this with regard to your problems, you can expect solutions.

But, you must set a limit to your desires. You must remember that the wealthy man is a man who is content with what he has. The happy man is the man who is content with what he is. This does not mean that you must remain in an inferior position. On the contrary, do whatever you can to advance, but do it without placing undue stress upon your health. The true happiness is to set goals within your reach. When you set a limit to your desires, set a limit to your ambition.

Learn to relax and enjoy life. Throughout these consultations you have been taught various methods to relax, and some that require limited forms of exercise such as the Buddha Walk and the Buddha Dance. The latter two combine relaxation with joy. When you practice these exercises you will be relaxing and experiencing the joy of living.

I would like to tell you the story—an ancient Zen story—of a man who was running away from a tiger. He came to the edge of a cliff with the tiger in hot pursuit and fell over the cliff. A few feet down, he grasped a branch of a bush that was growing from the cliff face. The tiger could not reach him. The man looked at the bush, and saw berries growing. He reached over, plucked a berry, put it in his mouth and said, "Oh, what a delicious berry."

There is a great lesson to be learned from this. There is still another lesson to be learned from the fact that when he looked down he saw tigers waiting in the valley below. Tigers above and tigers below. Worse still, a black and a white mouse were gnawing at the roots of the plant that was suspending him temporarily in the area of life, with death staring at him both above and below. The white and black mouse represent day and night, and as our nights and days pass, the fragile roots that hold us to life tear away. Death waits for us. But meanwhile, we must learn a lesson from this man! Reach over and pluck whatever berries you can, and say, "Oh, what delicious berries." You can only live NOW. Do it!

††*How Murray D. Used the EB—EB—EB Formulas for Happier Living*

You are now well acquainted with the famous empty bowel, empty bladder, empty brain formula. Look back at your eighth consultation for detailed information if you have forgotten. You will learn, or you now already know, that you must be able to empty your bowel, your bladder and your brain of self-destructive end products if you are to have better health. Murray was an unhappy man simply because he could never empty his bowel, his bladder or his brain of their troublesome contents. He had difficulty urinating as a result of an enlarged prostrate, difficulty emptying his bowel because he had developed a laxative habit over the years and difficulty emptying his brain simply because he did not know how. He was constantly worrying about what had happened in the past, living it over and over again with great regret, and he was in a state of total anxiety about the future. He never really lived in the present.

Obviously, this man could not be happy. Equally obviously, the solution to his problem is to be found in these consultations. He consulted me when he was in his early forties and began practicing the formulas you have learned to attain the empty bowel, empty bladder and empty brain. His prostate yielded at the same time that he learned to empty his bowel with the proper level of bran. As the pressure of the stool in his bowel was released, the prostate circulation improved, and this combined with the total Revitalization Plan, gave Murray D. a healthier bladder function, a healthier bowel function and a capacity for relaxation and reprogramming of his brain for happier living.

He learned to think positively. He learned to enjoy the present moment. He even learned to give his full attention to the master gland at the base of his brain—the pituitary gland—and learned this so well that he achieved deep relaxation at practically hibernation level that gave him the effect of eight hours of sleep during eight minutes of such relaxation. Indeed, Murray D. was one of my best students and most successful patients, and now—in his early seventies—is a very vital, very energetic, very happy man who lives one heartbeat, one moment, one day at a time.

More Food for the Body and the Mind

The soybean protein is a very high quality food. It contains practically the same food value as animal protein such as that in fish, meat, milk and eggs. The soybean protein is very high in essential amino acids that are the building blocks for normal cells, tissues and organs. Of all vegetables, the soybean is the best source of protein. Soybeans are also low in starch and sugar but very high in iron, calcium and phosphorus. In soybean oil there is vitamin A and D as well as E and K. And—as you now know—the oil is rich in unsaturated fatty acids.

The lecithin in the soybean is important for its unsaturated nature, for the fact that it helps in the ridding of deposits of saturated fats and cholesterol in the body, particularly in the arteries, and also because it contains phosphorus and choline. Phosphorus and choline are essential to the body, and you have already heard a great deal about lecithin in terms of the Revitalization Cocktail.

Sprouted soybeans not only offer a fine, tasty protein food, but also give you vitamin B-complex and a large amount of vitamin C. It is also claimed that sprouting soybeans have an increased amount of vitamin A as well as riboflavin and niacin.

If you are allergic to cow's milk, you can use soy milk in place of the skimmed milk in your Revitalization Cocktail. You will recall that I have offered the possibility of using skimmed milk as a base rather than orange juice, if you so desire. I now extend this for those of you who are allergic to cow's milk, and offer soy milk as a base in the Revitalization Cocktail.

For those of you who are looking for a less expensive coffee substitute, now that coffee is not only dangerous for its caffeine content, but it becoming increasingly expensive, you may wish to use heavily roasted and ground soybeans. They do not taste or smell like coffee, but may be obtained in powder form and will dissolve in hot water. There are other preparations of soy beverages for drip, percolator or silex coffee makers.

Other valuable beans include green beans and dry beans. Green beans contain vitamin A, the B vitamins and some vitamin C. Dry beans contain about three times the amount of the B vitamins as in green beans, though dry beans have no vitamin C, and less vitamin A.

Simple Formulations for Daily Use

The revitalized mind-body is a mind-body full of energy, great vitality and the capacity to enjoy life. That type of mind-body does not carry the problems of the past with it. Of course, it is sometimes necessary to review difficult, as yet unsolved problems, so that you may find the proper solution. But, once they are solved, they should be dropped from the mind. And, of course, those problems to which there is no solution should not be constantly dwelled upon. This does nothing but waste energy and lose vitality.

I am reminded of another ancient Zen story in which two monks were walking toward a stream. Buddhist monks are not even allowed to touch women. However, when they came to the edge of the stream they saw a woman who needed to cross the stream, but was obviously in great fear of the moving waters. One of the monks promptly bent down, took her upon his shoulders, and walked across the stream. When they came to the other side he put her down, and the two monks went on their way. As they walked, however, the monk who had carried the woman saw his brother monk looking at him with glances of disapproval. After a time the monk who had carried the woman turned to his companion and said, "You are still carrying her, aren't you?"

Here, too, we learn a great lesson from the Zen Master. You

must not carry the burdens of the past as you move on into the present and the future. What you must do is give your total attention to the present moment. Otherwise, you will not be living, but merely existing. The present moment may be a time of anxiety or a time of pleasure. It may be a time in which you are surrounded by great beauty, or a time in which you must work out a difficult problem. No matter what, you must give your full attention to the present moment before moving on.

And when you move on, you must leave the present moment behind, and once again give your attention to a new present moment. The past is dead. Bury it, instantly. The future is as yet unborn. You can only live *now*. I leave you with these words, but want to remind you once again that I am with you at all times if you wish me to be. As long as you have this book, you can refer back as often as you wish to my suggestions and my instructions. I am with you physically, in this book. I am with you in spirit at all times. May your life be happy, healthy and long. May you enjoy every moment of it.

††Your Instructions for Today. . .

1. **Practice the Buddha Walk at least once each day to loosen stiff joints and aching muscles.**
2. **Practice the Buddha Dance for renewed energy, lung and muscle strength.**
3. **Practice the half hour flexercise routine before bedtime, and combine this with the appropriate, "Better and better, happier and happier, healthier and healthier," for restful—usually dreamless sleep.**

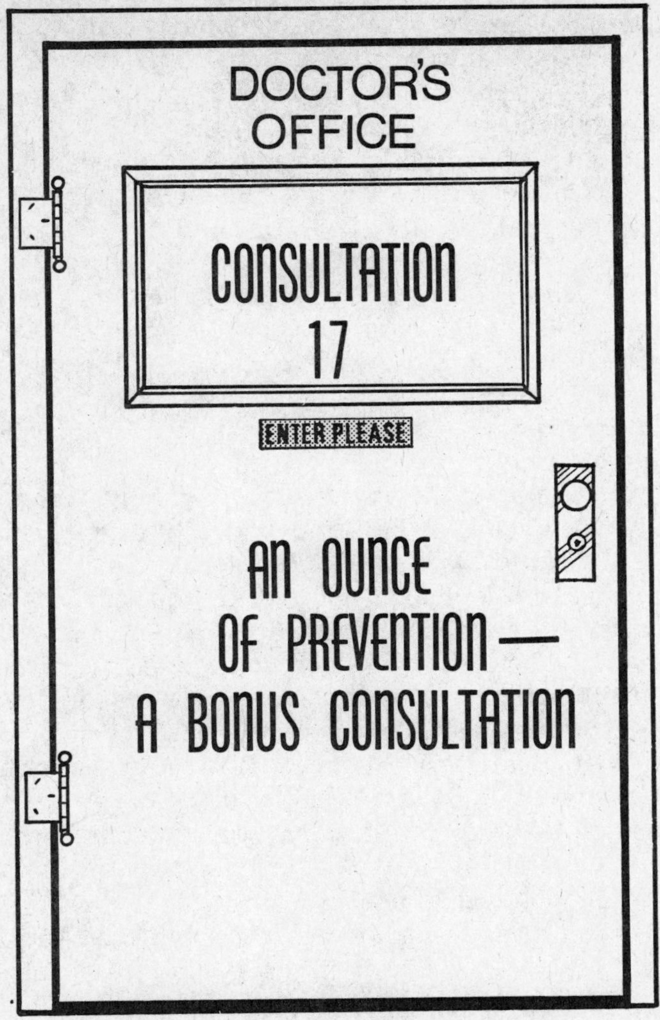

DOCTOR'S
OFFICE
CONSULTATION
17
ENTER PLEASE
AN OUNCE
OF PREVENTION—
A BONUS CONSULTATION

This is your bonus consultation—a most important bonus that may save your life. Remember the wise admonition—"An ounce of prevention is worth a pound of cure." Throughout these consultations, I have been offering you the ounce of prevention, as well as the added bonus of revitalization. Now, I will review and tell you still more about the ounce of prevention you can take to avoid one of the most dreaded diseases—cancer.

Let me begin with the need for regular rectal examination, to avoid cancer of the large bowel—the colon and rectum. If you are bleeding with bowel movement, the most likely cause will be varicose veins in the rectum—hemorrhoids (piles). But, since a change in your bowel habit and/or bleeding may be due to a more serious disease, if you experience a change, or bleeding, it is safest to immediately arrange for an examination with a lighted tube (a sigmoidscope) or with a fiberoptic and much longer tube (a colonoscope).

If your physician finds a polyp, it should be removed. Some polyps become malignant. If your doctor finds a cancer, he should take a specimen (a biopsy). This is a painless procedure. You should then be referred to a specialist in bowel cancer. Prevention is the better part of cure, and the removal of not-yet-malignant polyps is the ounce of prevention.

Wrong diet is among the primary causes of bowel cancer. We have already discussed this, but I must stress it once again. You already know about the work of Dr. Burkitt and his theory that a high fiber content in your food will reduce your chances of developing bowel cancer. The Revitalization Cocktail and Program provide this high fiber content—again your ounce of prevention. You will, at the same time, correct your constipation, perhaps prevent poylp formation and revitalize your entire body by avoiding refined sugars, processed starches and other supermarket high-sugar-content cereals with their additives.

There is much evidence to show that cancer of the bowel may be caused by a high saturated fat diet. Your Revitalization Cocktail contains polyunsaturated fat in limited quantity. Vitamin E to prevent free radical formation is part of your total Revitalization Program. You will also be avoiding saturated fats in steaks, other beef cuts, egg yolks, most cheese and butter when you follow the Revitalization Program. At the same time, you will be guarding your body against cardiovascular disease.

The proof of this "pudding" is in the statistics showing that Japanese who migrate to Hawaii and begin eating beef as we Americans do, have a higher incidence of bowel cancer than those who remain in Japan and eat little or no beef. I have friends who are Seventh Day Adventists and who do not eat meat. Those who are true vegetarians succumb to much fewer cancers of the bowel than the average high beef-eating Americans. Put the hamburger fast food stands out of bounds! The same results were found by

Dr. Michael Hill in England. A high-fat diet is somehow related to bowel cancer.

There is a comparable relationship between a high-fat diet and breast cancer! Women who are extremely overweight are even more susceptible to breast cancer.

Cancer of the tube leading from the mouth to the stomach (the esophagus), seems to be caused chiefly by cigarettes and alcohol. This combination is very deadly, and if you really want to revitalize yourself, you must absolutely give up both cigarettes and alcohol. You must also give up cigars and pipes if you inhale the smoke. Of course, the more you smoke and the more you drink alcoholic beverages, the greater the chance that you will develop cancer of the esophagus. Alcohol is also closely related to cancer of the mouth and throat, the voice box (larynx) and even cancer of the liver. The more you drink, the greater the destruction of your revitalization potential and the greater the likelihood that you will develop cancer. This is especially true if you are also a heavy smoker.

Liver cancer seems to occur especially in areas where there is a lack of protein in the diet. A fungus-produced poison called "aflatoxin" may cause such liver cancer, especially in Asia and Africa. In the United States liver cancer is quite rare in terms of aflatoxin.

You must also avoid smoked foods such as steaks broiled over charcoal (barbecue cancer) and roasted coffee, for these contain a cancer-causing chemical called benze(a)pyrene. Wherever smoking of food is common, as in Iceland, stomach cancer is also common. You will note that there are no such foods allowed in your Revitalization Program.

The Revitalization Program does not allow food additives, preservatives, dyes and so forth. You have already been instructed to avoid frankfurters, hamburgers, sausages, cold cuts and bacon, since they all contain a preservative called "nitrate." Your body combines the nitrates with amines from proteins in your food to produce the cancer-causing "nitrosamines." Remove such foods from your diet and you not only revitalize your body, but reduce your chances of cancer death. Revitalization and longevity will be your ounce of prevention bonus—your "pound of cure."

Our Food and Drug Administration has already banned certain cancer-causing dyes such as butter yellow and red dye. Others have been banned, but there are no doubt still many more to be researched and banned. Your lesson for today is to avoid artificially colored foods of all kinds.

Caffeine is definitely related to heart and artery disease. It may even be related to cancer in an indirect way,* but this is not yet certain. To be safe, eliminate caffeine from your diet, and don't forget that you will find it in tea, cocoa and cola drinks. Stay with bottled mineral waters (hard waters) from safe areas, fruit juices and skimmed milk as your regular beverages.

If you smoke, the Revitalization Program requires you to break this habit. Following is a condensation of an article taken from *Chest* magazine by permission about questions patients ask doctors which was written by Donald T. Fredrickson, M.D., Project Director, Inter-society Commission for Heart Disease Resources, New York, New York.[1]

Cigarette Smoking: Questions Patients Ask Doctors[1]

Smokers often raise challenging questions while trying to break the cigarette habit. Here are responses to some of these inquiries that may be helpful:

Question: Should I try to taper off gradually or stop suddenly?

Answer: Of the many who have been successful in stopping smoking, 50 percent report they stopped suddenly and 50 percent report they stopped gradually. In other words, both methods work and the "right way" to stop smoking is the way that is right for you. I would suggest gradual tapering off as a starter. This will give you small successes that will help restore confidence in your ability to manage the problem. In addition, gradual withdrawal will prepare you psychologically for that time when you are ready to make a bona fide decision to stop completely. Keep in mind, however, that there are certain smokers who find it extremely difficult to taper off. You may be one of these. If you are, set a date for stopping completely and prepare yourself for this. Remove all visible signs of the cigarette habit (cigarette packages, ashtrays, lighters, matches, holders) from your home and office. Store up on temporary substitutes—low-calorie candies, gum,

*Cancer of the female breast, and perhaps cancer of the prostate.

[1]Condensed from an article in *Chest*, Vol. 58, 1970.

thinly sliced strips of celery, carrots and so on. Prepare a three-day schedule filled with constant and intense activities; there should be virtually no time to sit around thinking about the fact that you are not smoking. During this period, you may or may not experience psychologic distress. If you do, you will find the critical period is the first 48 hours. Once beyond this point you will be well on your way towards meeting your goal of becoming a permanent nonsmoker.

Question: Why do I get so nervous when I try to stop smoking?

Answer: You use cigarettes to reduce uncomfortable feelings like the psychologic distress of anxiety, tension, anger, fear, boredom and so on. You will have to handle these feelings full force without the cigarette tranquilizer. For the great majority of smokers, the nervousness is temporary and begins to subside within a matter of days or at the most within a week or so.

Question: How long will the craving or urge to smoke last?

Answer: The craving to smoke is also temporary. Most successful ex-smokers report that within a matter of days the acute craving begins to subside and that, after two or three weeks there is only an occasional desire to light up.

Question: What about the physical symptoms I experience when I try to stop smoking? What causes these? Are they dangerous? How long will they last?

Answer: Examples of symptoms frequently reported are: nervousness, shortness of breath, tightness in the chest, heart palpitations, visual disturbances, sweats, abdominal discomfort, headaches, dizziness, fatigue, sleep disturbances, difficulty concentrating and short temper. The smoker should look upon these symptoms as a sign that he is successfully adjusting to the nonsmoking state. Most symptoms begin to subside within a matter of days or, at the most, within a week or so after stopping.

Symptoms associated with smoking withdrawal are not dangerous and need not be cause for alarm. Should symptoms persist for an inordinate period, the patient should be advised to consult his physician. Such symptoms may be totally unrelated to smoking cessation. Many smokers experience few, if any, physical or psychologic symptoms during withdrawal from cigarettes.

Question: Do you recommend switching to a pipe or cigar?

Answer: Because pipe and cigar smoke as a rule are not inhaled, these forms of tobacco constitute *less* of an overall hazard than cigarette smoking, I have little hesitancy in suggesting the transfer to cigars or a pipe if the smoker feels he must have a substitute or considers the switch a necessary step towards complete cessation. However, the smoker should be cautioned that if he switches to cigars or a pipe and continues to inhale he is certainly no better off for having made the transfer. In my experience heavy cigarette smokers who take up cigars or a pipe stay with these substitutes for a short period and then either stop completely or revert to cigarette smoking.

Question: Is there a filter that makes smoking safe?

Answer: Certain filters appear to give some protection against the hazards of cigarette smoking, especially those hazards (e.g., carcinoma of the lung) that have been associated with particulate matter in smoke. However, the degree of this protection has as yet to be determined. It should also be noted that there are many chemicals in tobacco smoke that are unaffected or only minimally affected by filters. To the extent that these cause illness, filters will have no protective value. The use of filtered cigarettes should never be used as a justification to continue smoking cigarettes.

Question: Is smoking an addiction? Am I like a drug addict?

Answer: Addiction refers to an alteration in the body's biochemistry, resulting from exposure to a drug. There is little evidence that basic alterations of this nature play any significant role in cigarette smoking. Rather, cigarette smoking can best be viewed as a habit—a form of behavior that is learned and consequently behavior subject to modification through a program of systematic relearning.

Question: What if I should backslide?

Answer: An episode of backsliding is no reason to feel defeated. One of the characteristics of learning a new habit is the tendency to temporarily fall back into the old familiar patterns of reacting. Every day you remain free of cigarettes will increase your chances of not succumbing to the temptation to smoke and, with time, the desire to smoke will lessen and eventually disappear altogether.

If perchance you should find yourself smoking again—don't panic. Remember, you have a lot going for you! When you've been free of cigarettes, even for a short period, considerable change has taken place within you. Stopping once again, provided you begin immediately, will not be nearly as difficult as it was before. Above all, never use an episode of backsliding as an excuse to start smoking again. If you backslide, you are faced with a critical decision—a decision you cannot avoid making. Either you are a smoker or you are on your way to becoming a non-smoker. Your job is to make the right decision!

Question: Will there be any immediate benefits if I stop smoking?

Answer: Smokers frequently report dramatic changes in their physical and psychological well-being shortly after they've stopped smoking.

Question: I'll crack up if I quit smoking or maybe I'll become an alcoholic.

Answer: On the contrary! When you finally gain control over the cigarette habit you may experience an increased ability to manage other "problems of living" more effectively.

Question: What can I do to avoid gaining weight when I stop smoking?

Answer: Many who stop smoking do not gain weight. Indeed, some even lose weight during withdrawal from cigarettes. When weight gain occurs, it is usually minimal and certainly should not discourage any smoker who is serious about controlling and finally mastering his cigarette problem. My advice is to concentrate on one habit at a time.

Question: I've been smoking a long time. The damage is probably already done—Is it too late for me to stop?

Answer: Let's eliminate such false reasoning. Irrespective of how long or how much you have smoked, when you stop smoking, the destruction that is caused by cigarettes stops and, because of the body's amazing recuperative powers, much of the damaged tissue may be repaired and replaced. This can be truly exciting news for the smoker. The message is a simple one—no matter how long or how much you have been smoking cigarettes, it is a scientific fact that when you stop smoking your body will begin the process of repairing damaged tissue!

Question: Can you give me a plan to follow for breaking the cigarette habit?

Answer: To recapitulate—every smoker can conquer the cigarette habit irrespective of how addicted, how defeated or discouraged he may feel or how many times he has temporarily stopped only to "fall off the wagon." To succeed, one trains himself in non-smoking the same way that he was trained in smoking.

For Your Family Doctor

The information in these consultations is designed for your patients. You will note that they are advised to consult with you before changing their eating or living habits. The Revitalization Plan is based upon my experience during the past forty years of practice, as well as upon the medical literature, the most recent research papers available to me as an editor, author and founder-executive of the Academy of Psychosomatic Medicine, the International Academy of Proctology, the International Board of Proctology, and the American Journal of Proctology Gastroenterology and Nutrition. It is also based upon personal communications with the discoverer of ascorbic acid, the most eminent advocates of this substance (both Nobel Laureates) and with the leading researchers in the fields of nutrition and oncology. The psychosomatic advice is based almost entirely upon my own experience and the books I have written on this subject, both for the physician and the layman.

If you wish further references on nutrition and cardiovascular disease, I believe that the text of this name, written by a distinguished list of contributors and edited by Elaine B. Feldman, M.D., Appleton Century Crofts, 1976, will provide the most recent technical and clinical research findings.

As for oncology and immunology, these fields—especially the latter—are in a state of constant change. Much of the material in my own text is based upon recent textbooks and papers in these fields, but even more represents my own thinking and evaluation. Time may alter these opinions, as it will add to and alter the presently accepted findings of the most prestigious research institutes. These are some of the reasons why I advise readers, as often as possible throughout the text, to consult with their own doctor. *You* must make the final decisions, based upon your knowledge of the patient. No one else can do this as well, certainly not an author whose work—no matter how much ahead of its time it may be—must stand the test of current research.

I am pleased that my own *Longevity Diet* (Parker Publishing), although first published in 1967, has stood the test of time and still provides a program that is current and useful. I am grateful to the many physicians who have advocated this book for their patients, and hope that the present Revitalization Program will also be helpful to the physician and the patient.

APPENDIX

Reference Text On the Composition of Foods

The following pages will provide the reader with a sample of the best and most authoritative U.S. Government sponsored reference material on the composition of foods. If you have any questions regarding the food you ordinarily eat or provide for your family, and are not certain that you are within the limits described in my book, you may wish to obtain the complete text. Write to the U.S. Government Printing Office, Washington, D.C., re the Department of Agriculture book, "The Composition of Foods."

Remember—you are what you eat and what you think (as well as what you inhale, of course). To be certain that you are eating foods that will provide you with the best possible nutrition for all body cells, and help you in your personal program of revitalization or rejuvenation, these sample reference pages (and the complete book) will be of permanent and reliable value to you and your family.

TABLE 1.—COMPOSITION OF FOODS, 100 GRAMS, EDIBLE PORTION

[Numbers in parentheses denote values imputed—usually from another form of the food or from a similar food. Zero in parentheses indicates that the amount of a constituent probably is none or is too small to measure. Dashes denote lack of reliable data for a constituent believed to be present in measurable amount. Calculated values, as those based on a recipe, are not in parentheses]

Item No.	Food and description	Water	Food energy	Protein	Fat	Carbohydrate		Ash	Calcium	Phos-phorus	Iron	Sodium	Potas-sium	Vitamin A value	Thiamine	Ribo-flavin	Niacin	Ascorbic acid
						Total	Fiber											
(A)	(B)	(C)	(D)	(E)	(F)	(G)	(H)	(I)	(J)	(K)	(L)	(M)	(N)	(O)	(P)	(Q)	(R)	(S)
		Percent	*Calories*	*Grams*	*Grams*	*Grams*	*Grams*	*Grams*	*Milligrams*	*Milligrams*	*Milligrams*	*Milligrams*	*Milligrams*	*International units*	*Milligrams*	*Milligrams*	*Milligrams*	*Milligrams*
	Abalone:																	
1	Raw	75.8	98	18.7	0.5	3.4	0	1.6	37	191	2.4	—	—	—	0.18	0.14	—	—
2	Canned	80.2	80	16.0	.3	2.3	0	1.2	14	128	—	—	—		.12	—	—	—
3	**Acerola** (Barbados-cherry or West Indian cherry), raw, pulp and skin.	92.3	28	.4	.3	6.8	.4	.2	12	11	.2	8	83	—	.02	.06	0.4	[1] 1,300
4	**Acerola juice, raw**	94.3	23	.4	.3	4.8	.3	.2	10	9	.5	3	—	—	.02	.06	.4	[2] 1,600
5	**Albacore, raw** [3]	66.2	177	25.3	7.6	0	0	1.3	26	—	—	40	293	—	—	—	—	5
	Ale. See Beverages: Beer, item 394.																	
	Alewife:																	
6	Raw	74.4	127	19.4	4.9	0	0	1.5	—	218	—	—	—	—	—	—	—	—
7	Canned, solids and liquid	73.0	141	16.2	8.0	0	0	3.4	—	—	—	—	—	—	—	—	—	—
	Algae. See Seaweeds, items 2027–2031.																	
	Alimentary pastes. See Macaroni, Noodles, Pastinas, Spaghetti.																	
	Almonds:																	
8	Dried	4.7	598	18.6	54.2	19.5	2.6	3.0	234	504	4.7	4	773	0	.24	.92	3.5	Trace
9	Roasted and salted	.7	627	18.6	57.7	19.5	2.6	3.5	235	504	4.7	198	773	0	.05	.92	3.5	0
	Sugar-coated. See Candy, item 613.																	
10	**Almond meal, partially defatted**	7.2	408	39.5	18.3	28.9	2.3	6.1	424	914	8.5	7	1,400	0	.32	1.68	6.3	Trace
11	**Amaranth, raw**	86.9	36	3.5	.5	6.5	1.3	2.6	267	67	3.9	—	411	6,100	.08	.16	1.4	80
12	**Anchovy, pickled, with and without added oil, not heavily salted.**	58.6	176	19.2	10.3	.3	0	11.6	168	210	—	—	—	—	—	—	—	—
	Apples:																	
	Raw, commercial varieties: [4]																	
	Freshly harvested and stored:																	
13	Not pared	84.4	58	.2	.6	14.5	1.0	.3	7	10	.3	1	110	90	.03	.02	.1	4
14	Pared	85.1	54	.2	.3	14.1	.6	.3	6	10	.3	1	110	40	.03	.02	.1	2
	Freshly harvested:																	
15	Not pared	84.8	56	.2	.6	14.1	1.0	.3	7	10	.3	1	110	90	.03	.02	.1	7
16	Pared	85.3	53	.2	.3	13.9	.6	.3	6	10	.3	1	110	40	.03	.02	.1	4
	Stored:																	
17	Not pared	83.9	60	.2	.7	14.8	1.0	.4	7	10	.3	1	110	90	.03	.02	.1	3
18	Pared	84.8	55	.2	.3	14.4	.6	.3	6	10	.3	1	110	40	.03	.02	.1	2
	Canned. See Applesauce, items 28–29.																	
	Dehydrated, sulfured:																	
19	Uncooked	2.5	353	1.4	2.0	92.1	3.8	2.0	40	66	2.0	7	730	—	Trace	.06	.6	10
20	Cooked, with added sugar	79.6	76	.2	.3	19.6	.5	.3	6	10	.3	1	106	—	Trace	.01	.1	1
	Dried, sulfured:																	
21	Uncooked	24.0	275	1.0	1.6	71.8	3.1	1.6	31	52	1.6	5	569	—	.06	.12	.5	10
	Cooked:																	
22	Without added sugar	78.4	78	.3	.5	20.3	.9	.5	9	15	.5	1	162	—	.01	.03	.1	Trace
23	With added sugar	69.7	112	.3	.4	29.2	.8	.4	8	13	.4	1	144	—	.01	.03	.1	Trace
24	Frozen, sliced, sweetened, not thawed	75.1	93	.2	.1	24.3	.7	.3	5	6	.5	[5] 14	68	20	.01	.03	.2	7
25	**Apple brown betty**	64.5	151	1.6	3.5	29.7	.5	.7	18	22	.6	153	100	100	.06	.04	.4	1
26	**Apple butter**	51.6	186	.4	.8	46.8	1.1	.4	14	36	.7	2	252	0	.01	.02	.2	2
27	**Apple juice, canned or bottled**	87.8	47	.1	Trace	11.9	.1	.2	.6	9	.6	1	101	—	.01	.02	.1	1
	Applesauce, canned:																	
28	Unsweetened or artificially sweetened	88.5	41	.2	.2	10.8	.6	.3	4	5	.5	2	78	40	.02	.01	Trace	1
29	Sweetened	75.7	91	.2	.1	23.8	.5	.2	4	5	.5	2	65	40	.02	.01	Trace	1
	Apricots:																	
30	Raw	85.3	51	1.0	.2	12.8	.6	.7	17	23	.5	1	281	2,700	.03	.04	.6	10
31	Candied	12.0	338	.6	.2	86.5	.6	.7	—	—	—	—	—	—	—	—	—	—
	Canned, solids and liquid:																	
32	Water pack, with or without artificial sweetener	89.1	38	.7	.1	9.6	.4	.5	12	16	.3	1	246	1,830	.02	.02	.4	4
33	Juice pack	84.5	54	1.0	.2	13.6	.4	.7	17	23	.5	1	362	2,700	.03	.03	.5	6
	Sirup pack:																	
34	Light	81.9	66	.7	.1	16.8	.4	.5	11	15	.3	1	239	1,780	.02	.02	.4	4
35	Heavy	76.9	86	.6	.1	22.0	.4	.4	11	15	.3	1	234	1,740	.02	.02	.4	4
36	Extra heavy	72.9	101	.6	.1	26.0	.4	.4	11	15	.3	1	230	1,720	.02	.02	.3	4
	Dehydrated, sulfured, nugget-type and pieces:																	
37	Uncooked	3.5	332	5.6	1.0	84.6	3.8	5.3	86	139	5.3	33	1,260	14,100	Trace	.08	3.6	15
38	Cooked, fruit and liquid, sugar added	66.7	119	1.3	.2	30.5	.9	1.3	20	33	1.3	8	299	2,800	Trace	.02	.8	2
	Dried, sulfured:																	
39	Uncooked	25.0	260	5.0	.5	66.5	3.0	3.0	67	108	5.5	26	979	10,900	.01	.16	3.3	12

	Cooked, fruit and liquid:																	
40	Without added sugar	75.6	85	1.6	.2	21.6	1.0	1.0	22	35	1.8	8	318	3,000	Trace	.05	1.0	3
41	With added sugar	66.2	122	1.4	.1	31.4	.9	.9	19	31	1.6	7	278	2,600	Trace	.04	.9	2
42	Frozen, sweetened, not thawed	73.3	98	.7	.1	25.1	.6	.8	10	19	.9	4	229	1,680	.02	.04	.8	[8]28
43	**Apricot nectar**, canned (approx. 40% fruit) [4]	84.6	57	.3	.1	14.6	.2	.4	9	12	.2	Trace	151	950	.01	.01	.2	3
	Artichokes, globe or French:																	
44	Raw	85.5	([7])	2.9	.2	[5]10.6	2.4	.8	51	88	1.3	43	430	160	.08	.05	1.0	12
45	Cooked, boiled, drained	86.5	([7])	2.8	.2	[5]9.9	2.4	.6	51	69	1.1	30	301	150	.07	.04	.7	8
	Artichokes, Jerusalem. See Jerusalem-artichokes, item 1150.																	
	Asparagus:																	
46	Raw spears	91.7	26	2.5	.2	5.0	.7	.6	22	62	1.0	2	278	900	.18	.20	1.5	33
47	Cooked spears, boiled, drained	93.6	20	2.2	.2	3.6	.7	.4	21	50	.6	1	183	900	.16	.18	1.4	26
	Canned spears:																	
	Green:																	
	Regular pack:																	
48	Solids and liquid	93.6	18	1.9	.3	2.9	.5	1.3	18	43	1.7	[9]236	166	510	.06	.09	.8	15
49	Drained solids	92.5	21	2.4	.4	3.4	.8	1.3	19	53	1.9	[9]236	166	800	.06	.10	.8	15
50	Drained liquid	95.6	11	.8	Trace	2.4	Trace	1.2	15	24	1.4	[9]236	166	Trace	.06	.07	.8	15
	Special dietary pack (low-sodium):																	
51	Solids and liquid	94.7	16	2.0	.2	2.7	.5	.4	18	43	1.7	3	166	510	.06	.09	.8	15
52	Drained solids	93.6	20	2.6	.3	3.1	.7	.4	19	53	1.9	3	166	800	.06	.10	.8	15
53	Drained liquid	96.8	9	.8	Trace	2.0	Trace	.4	15	24	1.4	3	166	Trace	.06	.07	.8	15
	White (bleached):																	
	Regular pack:																	
54	Solids and liquid	93.3	18	1.6	.3	3.3	.5	1.5	15	33	.9	[9]236	140	50	.05	.06	.7	15
55	Drained solids	92.3	22	2.1	.5	3.6	.8	1.5	16	41	1.0	[9]236	140	80	.05	.06	.7	15
56	Drained liquid	95.4	11	.7	Trace	2.5	Trace	1.4	13	18	.7	[9]236	140	Trace	.05	.04	.7	15
	Special dietary pack (low-sodium):																	
57	Solids and liquid	95.0	16	1.4	.2	3.0	.5	.4	15	33	.9	4	140	50	.05	.06	.7	15
58	Drained solids	94.0	19	1.9	.2	3.5	.7	.4	16	41	1.0	4	140	80	.05	.06	.7	15
59	Drained liquid	97.2	8	.6	Trace	1.8	Trace	.4	13	18	.7	4	140	Trace	.05	.04	.7	15
	Frozen:																	
	Cuts and tips:																	
60	Not thawed	92.3	23	3.3	.2	3.6	.8	.6	23	66	1.3	2	239	850	.16	.14	1.2	25
61	Cooked, boiled, drained	92.5	22	3.2	.2	3.5	.8	.6	22	64	1.2	1	220	850	.14	.13	1.0	23
	Spears:																	
62	Not thawed	92.0	24	3.3	.2	3.9	.8	.6	23	69	1.2	2	259	780	.18	.15	1.3	29
63	Cooked, boiled, drained	92.2	23	3.2	.2	3.8	.8	.6	22	67	1.1	1	238	780	.16	.14	1.1	26
	Avocados, raw:																	
64	All commercial varieties [10]	74.0	167	2.1	16.4	6.3	1.6	1.2	10	42	.6	4	604	290	.11	.20	1.6	14
65	California, mainly Fuerte	73.6	171	2.2	17.0	6.0	1.5	1.2	10	42	.6	4	604	290	.11	.20	1.6	14
66	Florida	78.0	128	1.3	11.0	8.8	(1.5)	.9	10	42	.6	4	604	290	.11	.20	1.6	14
	Baby foods: [11]																	
	Cereals, precooked, dry, and other cereal products:																	
67	Barley, added nutrients	6.6	348	13.4	1.2	73.6	1.2	5.2	736	821	53.2	452	413	(0)	3.71	1.20	32.2	(0)
68	High protein, added nutrients	5.9	357	35.2	3.7	48.1	2.2	7.1	815	904	63.1	653	1,078	—	3.67	1.15	24.0	(0)
69	Mixed, added nutrients	6.5	368	15.2	2.9	70.6	1.1	4.8	820	741	56.4	470	345	—	3.15	1.35	22.3	(0)
70	Oatmeal, added nutrients	7.0	375	16.5	5.5	66.0	1.5	5.0	757	734	48.2	437	374	(0)	2.58	1.05	21.3	(0)
71	Rice, added nutrients	7.2	371	6.6	1.6	80.0	.5	4.6	858	646	50.2	530	208	(0)	2.56	1.24	19.7	(0)
72	Teething biscuit	5.6	378	11.1	2.3	78.0	.7	3.0	322	347	4.6	421	250	—	.47	.57	3.0	(0)
	Wheat. See Farina, instant-cooking: items 995–996.																	
	Desserts, canned:																	
73	Custard pudding, all flavors	76.5	100	2.3	1.8	18.6	.2	.8	64	62	.3	150	94	100	.02	.12	.1	1
74	Fruit pudding with starch base, milk and/or egg (banana, orange, or pineapple).	75.7	96	1.2	.9	21.6	.3	.6	27	34	.3	128	75	100	.03	.05	.1	3
	Dinners, canned:																	
	Cereal, vegetable, meat mixtures (approx. 2%–4% protein):																	
75	Beef noodle dinner	88.2	48	2.8	1.1	6.8	.3	1.1	12	29	.5	269	159	620	.02	.05	.5	2
76	Cereal, egg yolk, and bacon	84.7	82	2.9	4.9	6.6	.1	.9	29	60	.8	301	36	520	.05	.06	.4	—
77	Chicken noodle dinner	88.5	49	2.1	1.3	7.2	.1	.9	27	30	.3	297	42	800	.03	.06	.4	1
78	Macaroni, tomatoes, meat, and cereal	84.5	67	2.6	2.0	9.6	.3	1.3	21	35	.5	381	77	500	.14	.12	1.0	1
79	Split peas, vegetables, and ham or bacon	81.5	80	4.0	2.1	11.2	.2	1.2	29	79	.7	295	112	600	.08	.05	.5	1
80	Vegetables and bacon, with cereal	85.7	68	1.7	2.9	8.7	.4	1.0	17	28	.6	282	130	2,200	.07	.05	.6	1
81	Vegetables and beef, with cereal	87.0	56	2.7	1.6	7.6	.4	1.1	17	39	.8	307	143	2,800	.03	.04	.9	1
82	Vegetables and chicken, with cereal	87.8	52	2.1	1.4	7.7	.2	1.0	33	33	.4	307	55	1,000	.03	.04	.5	Trace
83	Vegetables and ham, with cereal	85.6	64	2.8	2.2	8.3	.3	1.1	25	42	.3	360	90	1,000	.08	.05	.5	3

[1] Average for fully ripened fruit grown in Florida, Puerto Rico, Hawaii; range is from 1,000 to 2,000 mg. per 100 grams. At firm-ripe stage, average is 1,900 mg.; range, 1,200 to 2,700 mg. At partially ripe stage, average is 2,500 mg.; range, 1,200 to 4,500 mg. See also Notes on Foods, p. 178.

[2] Average for juice from ripe fruit; range is from 1,000 to 2,200 mg. per 100 grams.

[3] Almost all of catch is canned as tuna.

[4] See Notes on Foods: p. 174 for Apples; p. 177 for item 43.

[5] Average weighted in accordance with commercial freezing practices. See also Notes on Foods, p. 177.

[6] Average weighted in accordance with commercial freezing practices. For products without added ascorbic acid, average is about 9 mg. per 100 grams; for those with added ascorbic acid, about 65 mg.

[7] Values may range from 9 Calories per 100 grams for freshly harvested raw artichokes to as many as 47 for stored product; the corresponding range for boiled artichokes is 8 to 44 Calories.

[8] A large proportion of the carbohydrate in the unstored product may be inulin, which is of doubtful availability. During storage, inulin is converted to sugars.

[9] Estimated average based on addition of salt in the amount of 0.6 percent of the finished product.

[10] Values weighted according to production, estimated as 90 percent from California, 10 percent from Florida.

[11] Values for items in this group apply to both strained and chopped (or junior) foods, unless otherwise specified.

TABLE 1.—COMPOSITION OF FOODS, 100 GRAMS, EDIBLE PORTION—Continued

[Numbers in parentheses denote values imputed—usually from another form of the food or from a similar food. Zero in parentheses indicates that the amount of a constituent probably is none or is too small to measure. Dashes denote lack of reliable data for a constituent believed to be present in measurable amount. Calculated values, as those based on a recipe, are not in parentheses]

Item No.	Food and description	Water	Food energy	Protein	Fat	Carbohydrate		Ash	Calcium	Phosphorus	Iron	Sodium	Potassium	Vitamin A value	Thiamine	Riboflavin	Niacin	Ascorbic acid
						Total	Fiber											
(A)	(B)	(C)	(D)	(E)	(F)	(G)	(H)	(I)	(J)	(K)	(L)	(M)	(N)	(O)	(P)	(Q)	(R)	(S)
		Percent	Calories	Grams	Grams	Grams	Grams	Grams	Milligrams	Milligrams	Milligrams	Milligrams	Milligrams	International units	Milligrams	Milligrams	Milligrams	Milligrams
	Baby foods [11]—Continued																	
	Dinners, canned—Continued																	
	Cereal, vegetable, meat mixtures (approx. 2%-4% protein)—Continued																	
84	Vegetables and lamb, with cereal	87.0	58	2.2	2.0	7.7	0.3	1.1	23	37	0.7	269	148	2,200	0.03	0.05	0.7	1
85	Vegetables and liver, with cereal	87.8	47	3.1	.4	7.8	.3	.9	17	57	2.7	236	162	4,700	.04	.37	1.6	3
86	Vegetables and liver, with bacon and cereal	87.2	57	2.4	1.9	7.5	.3	1.0	11	42	2.6	284	131	4,600	.03	.33	1.3	2
87	Vegetables and turkey, with cereal	88.9	44	2.1	.8	7.2	.2	1.0	22	26	.3	307	46	400	.01	.03	.4	1
	Meat or poultry (approx. 6%-8% protein):																	
88	Beef with vegetables	81.6	87	7.4	3.7	6.0	.2	1.3	13	84	1.2	304	113	1,100	.07	.17	1.6	2
89	Chicken with vegetables	79.6	100	7.4	4.6	7.2	.2	1.2	22	85	.9	265	71	1,000	.09	.15	1.6	2
90	Turkey with vegetables	81.3	86	6.7	3.2	7.6	.5	1.2	38	63	.6	348	122	1,000	.13	.13	1.8	2
91	Veal with vegetables	85.0	63	7.1	1.6	5.1	.2	1.2	11	71	.8	323	95	800	.08	.15	2.0	2
	Fruits and fruit products, with or without thickening, canned:																	
92	Applesauce	80.8	72	.2	.2	18.6	.5	.2	4	7	.4	6	64	40	.01	.02	.1	Trace
93	Applesauce and apricots	76.7	86	.3	.1	22.6	.5	.3	4	14	.3	(4)	105	600	.01	.02	.1	2
94	Bananas (with tapioca or cornstarch, added ascorbic acid), strained.	77.5	84	.4	.2	21.6	.1	.3	13	10	.2	29	118	70	.02	.02	.2	35
95	Bananas and pineapple (with tapioca or cornstarch).	78.5	80	.4	.1	20.7	.1	.3	20	12	.2	59	72	30	.01	.01	.1	2
96	Fruit dessert with tapioca (apricot, pineapple, and/or orange).	77.6	84	.3	.3	21.5	.2	.3	15	9	.4	53	73	450	.02	.01	.2	4
97	Peaches	78.1	81	.6	.2	20.7	.5	.4	6	14	.3	(4)	80	500	.01	.02	.7	3
98	Pears	82.2	66	.3	.1	17.1	1.0	.3	7	8	.2	4	62	30	.02	.02	.2	2
99	Pears and pineapple	81.5	69	.4	.2	17.6	.9	.3	7	12	.2	(4)	72	20	.03	.02	.2	2
100	Plums with tapioca, strained	74.8	94	.4	.2	24.3	.3	.3	5	12	.4	38	44	250	.01	.02	.2	2
101	Prunes with tapioca	76.7	86	.3	.2	22.4	.3	.4	7	21	.9	33	120	400	.02	.06	.4	4
	Meats, poultry, and eggs; canned:																	
	Beef:																	
102	Strained	80.3	99	14.7	4.0	(0)	(0)	1.0	8	127	2.0	228	183	—	.01	.16	3.5	0
103	Junior	75.6	118	19.3	3.9	(0)	(0)	1.4	8	163	2.5	283	242	—	.02	.20	4.3	0
104	Beef heart	81.1	93	13.5	3.8	.4	(0)	1.2	5	155	3.7	208	—	—	.06	.62	3.6	0
105	Chicken	77.2	127	13.7	7.6	(0)	(0)	1.5	—	129	1.9	263	96	—	.02	.16	3.5	0
106	Egg yolks, strained	70.0	210	10.0	18.4	.2	(0)	1.4	81	256	3.0	273	59	1,900	.12	.22	Trace	Trace
107	Egg yolks with ham or bacon	70.3	208	10.0	18.1	.3	(0)	1.3	71	185	2.8	313	82	1,900	.10	.23	5	—
	Lamb:																	
108	Strained	79.3	107	14.6	4.9	(0)	(0)	1.2	9	124	2.1	241	181	—	.02	.17	3.3	—
109	Junior	76.0	121	17.5	5.1	(0)	(0)	1.4	13	156	2.7	294	228	—	.02	.21	4.1	—
110	Liver, strained	79.7	97	14.1	3.4	1.5	(0)	1.3	6	182	5.6	253	202	24,000	.05	2.00	7.6	10
111	Liver and bacon, strained	77.0	123	13.7	6.6	1.3	(0)	1.4	6	157	4.2	302	192	22,000	.05	1.99	7.8	7
	Pork:																	
112	Strained	77.7	118	15.4	5.8	(0)	(0)	1.1	8	130	1.5	223	178	—	.19	.20	2.7	—
113	Junior	74.3	134	18.6	6.0	(0)	(0)	1.3	8	144	1.2	237	210	—	.23	.23	2.8	—
	Veal:																	
114	Strained	80.7	91	15.5	2.7	(0)	(0)	1.1	10	145	1.7	226	214	—	.03	.20	4.3	—
115	Junior	76.9	107	18.8	3.0	(0)	(0)	1.4	8	157	1.6	276	206	—	.03	.22	6.0	—
	Vegetables, canned:																	
116	Beans, green	92.5	22	1.4	.1	5.1	.8	.9	33	25	1.1	213	93	400	.02	.06	.3	3
117	Beets, strained	89.2	37	1.4	.1	8.3	.6	1.0	18	27	.7	212	228	20	.02	.03	.1	3
118	Carrots	91.5	29	.7	.1	6.8	.6	.9	23	21	.5	169	181	13,000	.02	.03	.4	3
119	Mixed vegetables, including vegetable soup	88.5	37	1.6	.3	8.5	.5	1.1	22	36	.9	272	170	4,700	.05	.04	.6	2
120	Peas, strained	85.5	54	4.2	.2	9.3	.8	.8	11	63	1.2	194	100	500	.08	.09	1.2	10
121	Spinach, creamed	88.1	43	2.3	.7	7.5	.4	1.4	64	63	.6	272	142	5,000	.02	.13	.3	6
122	Squash	92.1	25	.7	.1	6.2	.8	.9	24	17	.4	292	138	2,400	.02	.04	.3	8
123	Sweetpotatoes	82.3	67	1.0	.2	15.5	.5	1.0	16	34	.4	187	180	4,900	.04	.03	.4	8
124	Tomato soup, strained	83.4	54	1.9	.1	13.5	.2	1.1	24	52	.4	294	300	1,000	.05	.12	.7	3
	Bacon, cured:																	
125	Raw, slab or sliced	19.3	665	8.4	69.3	1.0	0	2.0	13	108	1.2	680	130	(0)	.36	.11	1.8	—
126	Cooked, broiled or fried, drained	8.1	611	30.4	52.0	3.2	0	6.3	14	224	3.3	1,021	236	(0)	.51	.34	5.2	—
127	Canned	16.7	685	8.5	71.5	1.0	0	2.3	15	92	1.4	—	—	(0)	.23	.10	1.5	—
	Bacon, Canadian:																	
128	Unheated	61.7	216	20.0	14.4	.3	0	3.6	12	180	3.0	1,891	392	(0)	.83	.22	4.7	—
129	Cooked, broiled or fried, drained	49.9	277	27.6	17.5	.3	0	4.7	19	218	4.1	2,555	432	(0)	.92	.17	5.0	—

	Baking powders: [13]																	
	Home use: [13]																	
	Sodium aluminum sulfate:																	
130	With monocalcium phosphate monohydrate	1.6	129	.1	Trace	31.2	Trace	—	1,932	2,904	—	10,953	150	(0)	(0)	(0)	(0)	(0)
131	With monocalcium phosphate monohydrate and calcium carbonate.	1.0	78	.1	Trace	18.9	Trace	—	5,778	1,452	—	11,618	—	(0)	(0)	(0)	(0)	(0)
132	With monocalcium phosphate monohydrate and calcium sulfate.	1.3	104	.1	Trace	25.1	Trace	—	6,320	1,560	—	10,000	—	(0)	(0)	(0)	(0)	(0)
133	Straight phosphate	1.6	121	.1	Trace	29.3	Trace	—	6,279	9,438	—	8,220	170	(0)	(0)	(0)	(0)	(0)
	Tartrate:																	
134	Cream of tartar, with tartaric acid	1.0	78	.1	Trace	18.9	Trace	—	0	0	0	7,300	3,800	(0)	(0)	(0)	(0)	(0)
	Special low-sodium preparations:																	
135	Commercial powder	2.2	172	.1	Trace	41.6	Trace	—	4,816	7,308	—	[14] 6	10,948	(0)	(0)	(0)	(0)	(0)
136	Noncommercial formula [15]	1.1	83	.1	Trace	20.1	Trace	—	—	—	—	—	20,729	(0)	(0)	(0)	(0)	(0)
	Commercial use:																	
	Pyrophosphate:																	
137	No additional leavening acid	1.4	109	.1	Trace	26.5	Trace	—	0	11,954	—	16,804	—	(0)	(0)	(0)	(0)	(0)
138	With monocalcium phosphate monohydrate	1.4	105	.1	Trace	25.5	Trace	—	900	12,245	—	16,210	—	(0)	(0)	(0)	(0)	(0)
139	With monocalcium phosphate monohydrate and calcium lactate.	1.3	103	.1	Trace	25.0	Trace	—	[16] 993	11,580	—	15,947	—	(0)	(0)	(0)	(0)	(0)
140	**Bamboo shoots, raw**	91.0	27	2.6	.3	5.2	.7	.9	13	59	.5	—	533	20	.15	.07	.6	4
	Bananas:																	
	Raw:																	
141	Common	75.7	85	1.1	.2	22.2	.5	.8	8	26	.7	1	370	190	.05	.06	.7	10
142	Red	74.4	90	1.2	.2	23.4	.4	.8	10	18	.8	1	370	400	.05	.04	.6	(10)
143	Dehydrated, or banana powder	3.	340	4.4	.8	88.6	2.0	3.2	32	104	2.8	4	1,477	760	.18	.24	2.8	7
	Bananas, baking type. See Plantain, item 1634.																	
	Barbados-cherry. See Acerola, item 3.																	
144	**Barbecue sauce**	80.9	91	1.5	6.9	8.0	.6	2.7	21	20	.8	815	174	360	.01	.01	.3	5
	Barley, pearled:																	
145	Light	11.1	349	8.2	1.0	78.8	.5	.9	16	189	2.0	3	160	(0)	.12	.05	3.1	(0)
146	Pot or Scotch	10.8	348	9.6	1.1	77.2	.9	1.3	34	290	2.7	—	296	(0)	.21	.07	3.7	(0)
147	**Barracuda, Pacific, raw**	75.4	113	21.0	2.6	0	0	1.3	—	—	—	—	—	—	—	—	—	—
	Basella. See Vinespinach, item 2408.																	
	Bass, black sea:																	
148	Raw	79.3	93	19.2	1.2	0	0	1.2	—	—	—	68	256	—	—	—	—	—
149	Cooked, baked, stuffed [17]	52.9	259	16.2	15.8	11.4	—	3.7	—	—	—	—	—	—	—	—	—	—
150	**Bass, smallmouth and largemouth, raw**	77.3	104	18.9	2.6	0	0	1.2	—	192	—	—	—	—	.10	.03	2.1	—
	Bass, striped:																	
151	Raw	77.7	105	18.9	2.7	0	0	1.2	—	212	—	—	—	—	—	—	—	—
152	Cooked, oven-fried [18]	60.8	196	21.5	8.5	6.7	—	2.5	—	—	—	—	—	—	—	—	—	—
153	**Bass, white, raw**	78.8	98	18.0	2.3	0	0	1.0	—	—	—	—	—	—	—	—	—	—
	Beans, broad. See Broadbeans, items 481–482.																	
	Beans, common, mature seeds, dry:																	
	White:																	
154	Raw	10.9	340	22.3	1.6	61.3	4.3	3.9	144	425	7.8	19	1,196	0	.65	.22	2.4	—
155	Cooked	69.0	118	7.8	.6	21.2	1.5	1.4	50	148	2.7	[4] 7	416	0	.14	.07	.7	0
	Canned, solids and liquid:																	
156	With pork and tomato sauce	70.7	122	6.1	2.6	19.0	1.4	1.6	54	92	1.8	463	210	130	.08	.03	.6	2
157	With pork and sweet sauce	66.4	150	6.2	4.7	21.1	1.7	1.6	63	114	2.3	380	—	—	.06	.04	.5	—
158	Without pork	68.5	120	6.3	.5	23.0	1.4	1.7	68	121	2.0	338	268	60	.07	.04	.6	2
	Red:																	
159	Raw	10.4	343	22.5	1.5	61.9	4.2	3.7	110	406	6.9	10	984	20	.51	.20	2.3	—
160	Cooked	69.0	118	7.8	.5	21.4	1.5	1.3	38	140	2.4	[4] 3	340	Trace	.11	.06	.7	—
161	Canned, solids and liquid	76.0	90	5.7	.4	16.4	.9	1.5	29	109	1.8	3	264	Trace	.05	.04	.6	—
162	Pinto, calico, and red Mexican, raw	8.3	349	22.9	1.2	63.7	4.3	3.9	135	457	6.4	10	984	—	.84	.21	2.2	—
163	Other, including black, brown, and Bayo, raw	11.2	339	22.3	1.5	61.2	4.4	3.8	135	420	7.9	25	1,038	30	.55	.20	2.2	—
	Beans, hyacinth. See Hyacinth-beans, items 1137–1138.																	
	Beans, lima:																	
	Immature seeds:																	
164	Raw	67.5	123	8.4	.5	22.1	1.8	1.5	52	142	2.8	2	650	290	.24	.12	1.4	29
165	Cooked, boiled, drained	71.1	111	7.6	.5	19.8	1.8	1.0	47	121	2.5	1	422	280	.18	.10	1.3	17
	Canned:																	
	Regular pack:																	
166	Solids and liquid	80.8	71	4.1	.3	13.4	1.3	1.4	26	67	2.4	[9] 236	222	130	.04	.04	.5	7
167	Drained solids	74.7	96	5.4	.3	18.3	1.8	1.3	28	70	2.4	[9] 236	222	190	.03	.05	.5	6
168	Drained liquid	93.3	20	1.3	Trace	3.9	Trace	1.5	22	60	2.3	[9] 236	222	Trace	.04	.03	.6	10
	Special dietary pack (low-sodium):																	
169	Solids and liquid	81.7	70	4.4	.3	12.9	1.2	.7	26	67	2.4	4	222	130	.04	.04	.5	7
170	Drained solids	75.6	95	5.8	.3	17.7	1.8	.6	28	70	2.4	4	222	190	.03	.05	.5	6
171	Drained liquid	94.4	19	1.4	Trace	3.5	Trace	.7	22	60	2.3	4	222	Trace	.04	.03	.6	10

[4] See Notes on Foods: p. 176 for items 155 and 160; p. 177 for items 93, 97, and 99.

[9] Estimated average based on addition of salt in the amount of 0.6 percent of the finished product.

[12] Values for energy and proximate constituents are based on starch content.

[13] List of ingredients on label indicates type of baking powder.

[14] Value based on single brand.

[15] Values are based on formula in "Planning Low-Sodium Meals," Newton Health Dept., Newton, Mass., 1951, as cited in National Academy of Sciences–National Research Council Publication No. 325 "Sodium-Restricted Diets," p. 20, 1954, Washington, D.C.

[16] Calcium content depends largely on amount of monocalcium phosphate in the product. Values range from 200 to 1,600 mg. per 100 grams.

[17] Prepared with bacon, butter, onion, celery, and bread cubes.

[18] Prepared with milk, bread crumbs, butter, and salt.

TABLE 1.—COMPOSITION OF FOODS, 100 GRAMS, EDIBLE PORTION—Continued

[Numbers in parentheses denote values imputed—usually from another form of the food or from a similar food. Zero in parentheses indicates that the amount of a constituent probably is none or is too small to measure. Dashes denote lack of reliable data for a constituent believed to be present in measurable amount. Calculated values, as those based on a recipe, are not in parentheses]

Item No.	Food and description	Water	Food energy	Protein	Fat	Carbohydrate		Ash	Calcium	Phosphorus	Iron	Sodium	Potassium	Vitamin A value	Thiamine	Riboflavin	Niacin	Ascorbic acid
						Total	Fiber											
(A)	(B)	(C)	(D)	(E)	(F)	(G)	(H)	(I)	(J)	(K)	(L)	(M)	(N)	(O)	(P)	(Q)	(R)	(S)
		Percent	Calories	Grams	Grams	Grams	Grams	Grams	Milligrams	Milligrams	Milligrams	Milligrams	Milligrams	International units	Milligrams	Milligrams	Milligrams	Milligrams
	Beans, lima—Continued																	
	Immature seeds—Continued																	
	Frozen:																	
	Thick-seeded types, commonly called Fordhooks:																	
172	Not thawed	72.7	102	6.2	0.1	19.5	1.7	1.5	23	96	1.9	[10]129	490	230	0.10	0.06	1.2	22
173	Cooked, boiled, drained	73.5	99	6.0	.1	19.1	1.6	1.3	20	90	1.7	101	426	230	.07	.05	1.0	17
	Thin-seeded types, commonly called baby limas:																	
174	Not thawed	67.8	122	7.6	.2	23.0	1.9	1.4	38	131	2.8	[10]147	438	220	.10	.06	1.2	19
175	Cooked, boiled, drained	68.8	118	7.4	.2	22.3	1.9	1.3	35	126	2.6	129	394	220	.09	.05	1.2	12
	Mature seeds, dry:																	
176	Raw	10.3	345	20.4	1.6	64.0	4.3	3.7	72	385	7.8	4	1,529	Trace	.48	.17	1.9	—
177	Cooked	64.1	138	8.2	.6	25.6	1.7	1.5	29	154	3.1	[4]2	612	—	.13	.06	.7	—
178	**Bean flour, lima**	10.5	343	21.5	1.4	63.0	2.	3.6	—	—	—	—	—	(0)	—	—	—	(0)
	Beans, mung:																	
179	Mature seeds, dry, raw	10.7	340	24.2	1.3	60.3	4.4	3.5	118	340	7.7	6	1,028	80	.38	.21	2.6	—
	Sprouted seeds:																	
180	Uncooked	88.8	35	3.8	.2	6.6	.7	.6	19	64	1.3	5	223	20	.13	.13	.8	19
181	Cooked, boiled, drained	91.0	28	3.2	.2	5.2	.7	.4	17	48	.9	4	156	20	.09	.10	.7	6
	Beans, snap:																	
	Green:																	
182	Raw	90.1	32	1.9	.2	7.1	1.0	.7	56	44	.8	7	243	600	.08	.11	.5	19
	Cooked, boiled, drained, cooked in—																	
183	Small amount of water, short time	92.4	25	1.6	.2	5.4	1.0	.4	50	37	.6	4	151	540	.07	.09	.5	12
184	Large amount of water, long time	92.4	25	1.6	.2	5.4	1.0	.4	50	37	.6	4	151	540	.06	.08	.3	10
	Canned:																	
	Regular pack:																	
185	Solids and liquid	93.5	18	1.0	.1	4.2	.6	1.2	34	21	1.2	[9]236	95	290	.03	.04	.3	4
186	Drained solids	91.9	24	1.4	.2	5.2	1.0	1.3	45	25	1.5	[9]236	95	470	.03	.05	.3	4
187	Drained liquid	95.9	10	.4	.1	2.4	Trace	1.2	15	14	.9	[9]236	95	Trace	.03	.03	.3	4
	Special dietary pack (low-sodium):																	
188	Solids and liquid	94.8	16	1.1	.1	3.6	.6	.4	34	21	1.2	2	95	290	.03	.04	.3	4
189	Drained solids	93.2	22	1.5	.1	4.8	.9	.4	45	25	1.5	2	95	470	.03	.05	.3	4
190	Drained liquid	97.3	8	.4	.1	1.8	Trace	.4	15	14	.9	2	95	Trace	.03	.03	.3	4
	Frozen:																	
	Cut:																	
191	Not thawed	91.7	26	1.7	.1	6.0	1.0	.5	42	33	.8	1	167	580	.07	.10	.4	9
192	Cooked, boiled, drained	92.1	25	1.6	.1	5.7	1.0	.5	40	32	.7	1	152	580	.07	.09	.4	5
	French style:																	
193	Not thawed	91.6	27	1.7	.1	6.1	1.1	.5	40	32	.9	2	153	530	.07	.09	.4	10
194	Cooked, boiled, drained	91.9	26	1.6	.1	6.0	1.1	.4	38	30	.9	2	136	530	.06	.08	.3	7
	Yellow or wax:																	
195	Raw	91.4	27	1.7	.2	6.0	1.0	.7	56	43	.8	7	243	250	.08	.11	.5	20
196	Cooked, boiled, drained	93.4	22	1.4	.2	4.6	1.0	.4	50	37	.6	3	151	230	.07	.09	.5	13
	Canned:																	
	Regular pack:																	
197	Solids and liquid	93.7	19	1.0	.2	4.2	.6	.9	34	21	1.2	[9]236	95	60	.03	.04	.3	5
198	Drained solids	92.2	24	1.4	.3	5.2	.9	.9	45	25	1.5	[9]236	95	100	.03	.05	.3	5
199	Drained liquid	96.1	11	.4	.1	2.5	Trace	.9	15	14	.9	[9]236	95	Trace	.03	.03	.3	5
	Special dietary pack (low-sodium):																	
200	Solids and liquid	95.2	15	.9	.1	3.4	.6	.4	(34)	(21)	(1.2)	2	95	(60)	(.03)	(.04)	(.3)	(5)
201	Drained solids	93.6	21	1.2	.1	4.7	.9	.4	(45)	(25)	(1.5)	2	95	(100)	(.03)	(.05)	(.3)	(5)
202	Drained liquid	97.7	7	.4	.1	1.4	Trace	.4	(15)	(14)	(.9)	2	95	Trace	(.03)	(.03)	(.3)	(5)
	Frozen, cut:																	
203	Not thawed	91.1	28	1.8	.1	6.5	1.1	.5	36	32	.8	1	180	100	.08	.09	.5	12
204	Cooked, boiled, drained	91.5	27	1.7	.1	6.2	1.1	.5	35	31	.7	1	164	100	.07	.08	.4	6
	Bean sprouts. See Beans, mung: items 180–181; and Soybeans: items 2143–2144.																	
205	**Beans and frankfurters, canned**	70.7	144	7.6	7.1	12.6	1.0	2.0	37	119	1.9	539	262	130	.07	.06	1.3	Trace
206	**Beaver**, cooked, roasted	56.2	248	29.2	13.7	0	0	.9	—	—	—	—	—	—	.08	.38	—	—
207	**Beechnuts**	6.6	568	19.4	50.0	20.3	3.7	3.7	—	—	—	—	—	—	—	—	—	—

No.	Food																	
	Beef: [4]																	
	Carcass:																	
	Total edible, including kidney and kidney fat, raw:																	
208	Prime grade (54% lean, 46% fat)	44.8	428	13.6	41.	0	0	.6	8	124	2.0			80	.06	.12	3.3	—
209	Choice grade (60% lean, 40% fat)	49.4	379	14.9	35.	0	0	.7	9	136	2.2			70	.06	.13	3.6	—
210	Good grade (66% lean, 34% fat)	54.7	323	16.5	28.	0	0	.8	10	152	2.5			60	.07	.15	4.0	—
211	Standard grade (73% lean, 27% fat)	60.1	266	18.0	21.	0	0	.9	10	166	2.7			40	.08	.16	4.3	—
212	Commercial grade (64% lean, 36% fat)	52.4	347	15.8	31.	0	0	.8	9	145	2.4			60	.07	.14	3.8	—
213	Utility grade (76% lean, 24% fat)	62.5	242	18.6	18.	0	0	.9	11	172	2.8			40	.08	.17	4.5	—
	Total edible, trimmed to retail level, raw:																	
214	Choice grade (75% lean, 25% fat)	56.7	301	17.4	25.1	0	0	.8	10	161	2.6			50	.07	.15	4.2	—
215	Good grade (78% lean, 22% fat)	60.3	263	18.5	20.4	0	0	.8	11	171	2.8			40	.08	.16	4.4	—
216	Standard grade (82% lean, 18% fat)	63.9	225	19.4	15.8	0	0	.9	11	180	2.9			30	.08	.17	4.7	—
	Separable fat:																	
	Raw. See individual cuts.																	
217	Cooked	15.7	729	5.7	78.1	0	0	.5	—	—	—			—	—	—	—	—
	Retail cuts, trimmed to retail level:																	
	Chuck cuts:																	
	Entire chuck, 1st–5th ribs, arm, and neck:																	
	Choice grade:																	
	Total edible:																	
218	Raw (82% lean, 18% fat)	60.8	257	18.7	19.6	0	0	.9	11	188	2.8			40	.08	.17	4.5	—
219	Cooked, braised or pot-roasted (81% lean, 19% fat).	49.4	327	26.0	23.9	0	0	.7	11	140	3.3			40	.05	.20	4.0	—
	Separable lean:																	
220	Raw	70.3	158	21.3	7.4	0	0	1.0	12	214	3.2			10	.09	.19	5.1	—
221	Cooked, braised or pot-roasted	59.7	214	30.0	9.5	0	0	.8	13	160	3.8			20	.05	.23	4.6	—
	Separable fat:																	
222	Raw	16.9	716	6.6	76.3	0	0	.2	4	72	1.0			150	.03	.06	1.6	—
	Chuck rib, 5th:																	
	Choice grade:																	
	Total edible:																	
223	Raw (70% lean, 30% fat)	51.7	352	16.2	31.4	0	0	.7	9	148	2.4			60	.07	.14	3.9	—
224	Cooked, braised (69% lean, 31% fat)	40.3	427	22.4	36.7	0	0	.6	10	110	2.9			70	.04	.17	3.5	—
	Separable lean:																	
225	Raw	67.4	188	20.7	11.0	0	0	.9	12	192	3.1			20	.09	.18	5.0	—
226	Cooked, braised	56.5	249	28.9	13.9	0	0	.7	13	143	3.7	([20])	([21])	20	.05	.22	4.5	—
	Separable fat:																	
227	Raw	14.3	745	5.5	80.0	0	0	.2	3	45	.8			160	.02	.05	1.3	—
	Good grade:																	
	Total edible:																	
228	Raw (74% lean, 26% fat)	56.3	303	17.5	25.3	0	0	.8	10	162	2.6			50	.08	.16	4.2	—
229	Cooked, braised (73% lean, 27% fat)	44.8	377	24.2	30.3	0	0	.7	10	121	3.1			60	.04	.19	3.8	—
	Separable lean:																	
230	Raw	69.8	163	21.2	8.0	0	0	1.0	12	197	3.2			20	.09	.19	5.1	—
231	Cooked, braised	59.2	219	29.8	10.2	0	0	.8	13	147	3.8			20	.05	.23	4.6	—
	Separable fat:																	
232	Raw	17.8	705	7.0	74.9	0	0	.3	4	60	1.0			150	.03	.06	1.7	—
	Arm:																	
	Choice grade:																	
	Total edible:																	
233	Raw (86% lean, 14% fat)	64.2	223	19.4	15.5	0	0	.9	12	180	2.9			30	.08	.17	4.7	—
234	Cooked, braised or pot-roasted (85% lean, 15% fat).	53.0	289	27.1	19.2	0	0	.7	12	134	3.4			30	.05	.21	4.2	—
	Separable lean:																	
235	Raw	72.0	141	21.6	5.4	0	0	1.0	13	201	3.2			10	.09	.19	5.2	—
236	Cooked, braised or pot-roasted	61.7	193	30.5	7.0	0	0	.8	14	150	3.8			10	.06	.23	4.6	—
	Separable fat:																	
237	Raw	15.2	736	5.8	78.8	0	0	.2	3	48	.9			160	.02	.05	1.4	—
	Good grade:																	
	Total edible:																	
238	Raw (89% lean, 11% fat)	67.3	191	20.3	11.6	0	0	.9	12	188	3.1			20	.09	.18	4.8	—
239	Cooked, braised or pot-roasted (88% lean, 12% fat).	56.3	253	28.4	14.6	0	0	.7	13	140	3.7			30	.05	.21	4.3	—
	Separable lean:																	
240	Raw	73.2	129	21.8	4.0	0	0	1.0	13	203	3.3			10	.09	.19	5.2	—
241	Cooked, braised or pot-roasted	63.1	179	30.9	5.2	0	0	.8	14	151	3.9			10	.06	.23	4.7	—
	Separable fat:																	
242	Raw	17.9	704	7.1	74.7	0	0	.3	4	61	1.1			150	.03	.06	1.7	—

[4] See Notes on Foods: p. 176 for item 177; p. 179 for Beef.

[9] Estimated average based on addition of salt in the amount of 0.6 percent of the finished product.

[19] Average weighted in accordance with commercial practices in freezing vegetables. See also Notes on Foods, p. 177.

[20] Average value for 100 grams, all cuts, is 65 mg. for raw beef and 60 mg. for cooked beef. See also Notes on Foods, p. 179.

[21] Average value per 100 grams of beef of all cuts is 355 mg. for raw meat and 370 mg. for cooked meat.

TABLE 1.—COMPOSITION OF FOODS, 100 GRAMS, EDIBLE PORTION—Continued

[Numbers in parentheses denote values imputed—usually from another form of the food or from a similar food. Zero in parentheses indicates that the amount of a constituent probably is none or is too small to measure. Dashes denote lack of reliable data for a constituent believed to be present in measurable amount. Calculated values, as those based on a recipe, are not in parentheses]

Item No.	Food and description	Water	Food energy	Protein	Fat	Carbohydrate		Ash	Calcium	Phosphorus	Iron	Sodium	Potassium	Vitamin A value	Thiamine	Riboflavin	Niacin	Ascorbic acid
						Total	Fiber											
(A)	(B)	(C)	(D)	(E)	(F)	(G)	(H)	(I)	(J)	(K)	(L)	(M)	(N)	(O)	(P)	(Q)	(R)	(S)
		Percent	Calories	Grams	Grams	Grams	Grams	Grams	Milligrams	Milligrams	Milligrams	Milligrams	Milligrams	International units	Milligrams	Milligrams	Milligrams	Milligrams
	Beef[4]—Continued																	
	Retail cuts, trimmed to retail level—Continued																	
	Flank steak:																	
	Choice grade:																	
	Total edible:																	
243	Raw (100% lean)	71.7	144	21.6	5.7	0	0	1.0	13	201	3.2			10	0.09	0.19	5.2	—
244	Cooked, braised (100% lean)	61.4	196	30.5	7.3	0	0	.8	14	150	3.8			10	.06	.23	4.6	—
	Good grade:																	
	Total edible:																	
245	Raw (100% lean)	72.1	139	21.8	5.1	0	0	1.0	13	203	3.3			10	.09	.19	5.2	—
246	Cooked, braised (100% lean)	61.8	191	30.8	6.6	0	0	.8	14	151	3.9			10	.06	.23	4.7	—
	Hindshank:																	
	Choice grade:																	
	Total edible:																	
247	Raw (67% lean, 33% fat)	57.6	289	18.2	23.4	0	0	.8	11	168	2.8			50	.08	.16	4.4	—
248	Cooked, simmered (66% lean, 34% fat)	46.1	361	25.1	28.1	0	0	.7	11	125	3.3			50	.05	.19	3.9	—
	Separable lean:																	
249	Raw	72.7	134	21.7	4.6	0	0	1.0	13	202	3.3			10	.09	.19	5.2	—
250	Cooked, simmered	62.5	184	30.7	5.9	0	0	.8	14	151	3.9			10	.06	.23	4.7	—
	Separable fat:																	
251	Raw	27.0	602	11.1	61.5	0	0	.4	6	100	1.7			120	.05	.10	2.7	—
	Good grade:																	
	Total edible:																	
252	Raw (71% lean, 29% fat)	62.3	239	19.7	17.2	0	0	.8	12	182	3.0			30	.08	.17	4.7	—
253	Cooked, simmered (70% lean, 30% fat)	51.0	307	27.2	21.1	0	0	.7	12	136	3.6			40	.05	.21	4.2	—
	Separable lean:																	
254	Raw	73.5	126	21.8	3.7	0	0	1.0	13	203	3.3			10	.09	.19	5.2	—
255	Cooked, simmered	63.4	176	31.0	4.8	0	0	.8	14	151	3.9			10	.06	.23	4.7	—
	Separable fat:																	
256	Raw	34.6	517	14.5	50.4	0	0	.5	8	132	2.2			100	.06	.13	3.5	—
	Loin or short loin:																	
	Porterhouse steak:																	
	Choice grade:																	
	Total edible:											(30)	(31)					
257	Raw (63% lean, 37% fat)	48.3	390	14.8	36.2	0	0	.7	8	136	2.2			70	.06	.13	3.6	—
258	Cooked, broiled (57% lean, 43% fat)	37.2	465	19.7	42.2	0	0	.9	9	168	2.6			70	.06	.16	4.2	—
	Separable lean:																	
259	Raw	69.7	164	21.1	8.2	0	0	1.0	12	196	3.2			20	.09	.19	5.1	—
260	Cooked, broiled	57.9	224	30.2	10.5	0	0	1.4	12	242	3.7			20	.08	.23	5.9	—
	Separable fat:																	
261	Raw	11.5	777	4.2	84.1	0	0	.2	2	33	.6			170	.02	.04	1.0	—
	Good grade:																	
	Total edible:																	
262	Raw (64% lean, 36% fat)	50.2	370	15.3	33.8	0	0	.7	8	140	2.3			70	.06	.14	3.7	—
263	Cooked, broiled (58% lean, 42% fat)	38.9	446	20.5	39.7	0	0	1.0	9	173	2.6			70	.06	.17	4.3	—
	Separable lean:																	
264	Raw	72.0	141	21.5	5.5	0	0	1.0	12	200	3.2			10	.09	.19	5.2	—
265	Cooked, broiled	60.3	197	31.1	7.1	0	0	1.4	12	247	3.7			10	.08	.24	6.0	—
	Separable fat:																	
266	Raw	11.6	775	4.3	83.9	0	0	.2	2	34	.6			170	.02	.04	1.0	—
	T-bone steak:																	
	Choice grade:																	
	Total edible:																	
267	Raw (62% lean, 38% fat)	47.5	397	14.7	37.1	0	0	.7	8	135	2.2			70	.06	.13	3.5	—
268	Cooked, broiled (56% lean, 44% fat)	36.4	473	19.5	43.2	0	0	.9	8	166	2.6			80	.06	.16	4.1	—
	Separable lean:																	
269	Raw	69.7	164	21.2	8.1	0	0	1.0	12	197	3.2			20	.09	.19	5.1	—
270	Cooked, broiled	57.9	223	30.4	10.3	0	0	1.4	12	243	3.7			20	.08	.23	5.9	—
	Separable fat:																	
271	Raw	11.7	774	4.3	83.8	0	0	.2	2	34	.6			170	.02	.04	1.0	—
	Good grade:																	
	Total edible:																	
272	Raw (64% lean, 36% fat)	50.6	366	15.4	33.3	0	0	.7	9	142	2.3			70	.07	.14	3.7	—
273	Cooked, broiled (58% lean, 42% fat)	39.2	442	20.6	39.2	0	0	1.0	9	175	2.7			70	.06	.17	4.3	—

	Separable lean:																	
274	Raw	71.9	142	21.5	5.6	0	0	1.0	12	200	3.2			10	.09	.19	5.2	—
275	Cooked, broiled	60.2	199	31.1	7.3	0	0	1.4	12	247	3.7			10	.08	.24	6.0	—
	Separable fat:																	
276	Raw	12.9	761	4.8	82.1	0	0	.2	3	39	.7			160	.02	.04	1.2	—
	Club steak:																	
	Choice grade:																	
	Total edible:																	
277	Raw (64% lean, 36% fat)	49.1	380	15.5	34.8	0	0	.7	9	142	2.3			70	.07	.14	3.7	—
278	Cooked, broiled (58% lean, 42% fat)	37.9	454	20.6	40.6	0	0	.9	9	175	2.7			70	.06	.17	4.3	—
	Separable lean:																	
279	Raw	67.9	182	20.8	10.3	0	0	1.0	12	193	3.1			20	.09	.19	5.0	—
280	Cooked, broiled	56.0	244	29.6	13.0	0	0	1.4	12	238	3.6			20	.08	.23	5.8	—
	Separable fat:																	
281	Raw	15.6	731	6.0	78.2	0	0	.2	3	50	.9			160	.03	.05	1.4	—
	Good grade:																	
	Total edible:																	
282	Raw (70% lean, 30% fat)	54.5	324	16.9	27.9	0	0	.8	10	156	2.6			60	.07	.15	4.0	—
283	Cooked, broiled (64% lean, 36% fat)	42.8	398	22.9	33.3	0	0	1.0	10	192	3.0			60	.06	.18	4.7	—
	Separable lean:																	
284	Raw	70.3	158	21.2	7.5	0	0	1.0	12	197	3.2			20	.09	.19	5.1	—
285	Cooked, broiled	58.5	217	30.5	9.6	0	0	1.4	12	243	3.7			20	.08	.23	5.9	—
	Separable fat:																	
286	Raw	17.0	716	6.6	76.2	0	0	.2	4	56	1.0			150	.03	.06	1.6	—
	Loin end or sirloin:																	
	Wedge and round-bone sirloin steak:																	
	Choice grade:																	
	Total edible:																	
287	Raw (73% lean, 27% fat)	55.7	313	16.9	26.7	0	0	.8	10	155	2.5			50	.07	.15	4.1	—
288	Cooked, broiled (66% lean, 34% fat)	43.9	387	23.0	32.0	0	0	1.1	10	191	2.9			50	.06	.18	4.7	—
	Separable lean:																	
289	Raw	71.8	143	21.5	5.7	0	0	1.0	12	200	3.2			10	.09	.19	5.2	—
290	Cooked, broiled	58.7	207	32.2	7.7	0	0	1.5	13	261	3.9			10	.09	.25	6.4	—
	Separable fat:																	
291	Raw	11.8	773	4.4	83.6	0	0	.2	3	35	.7			170	.02	.04	1.1	—
	Good grade:																	
	Total edible:																	
292	Raw (75% lean, 25% fat)	58.7	281	17.8	22.7	0	0	.8	10	164	2.7			50	.08	.16	4.3	—
293	Cooked, broiled (68% lean, 32% fat)	46.9	353	24.5	27.5	0	0	1.1	11	202	3.1	(30)	(31)	50	.07	.19	5.0	—
	Separable lean:																	
294	Raw	73.2	129	21.8	4.0	0	0	1.0	13	203	3.3			10	.09	.19	5.2	—
295	Cooked, broiled	61.6	183	31.7	5.3	0	0	1.4	13	250	3.8			10	.08	.24	6.1	—
	Separable fat:																	
296	Raw	14.4	744	5.5	79.9	0	0	.2	3	45	.8			160	.02	.05	1.3	—
	Double-bone sirloin steak:																	
	Choice grade:																	
	Total edible:																	
297	Raw (72% lean, 28% fat)	53.7	333	16.4	29.1	0	0	.8	9	151	2.5			60	.07	.15	3.9	—
298	Cooked, broiled (66% lean, 34% fat)	42.1	408	22.2	34.7	0	0	1.0	10	186	2.9			60	.06	.18	4.6	—
	Separable lean:																	
299	Raw	70.3	158	21.3	7.4	0	0	1.0	12	198	3.2			20	.09	.19	5.1	—
300	Cooked, broiled	58.5	216	30.6	9.5	0	0	1.4	12	244	3.7			20	.08	.23	6.0	—
	Separable fat:																	
301	Raw	10.1	793	3.6	86.2	0	0	.1	2	27	.5			170	.02	.03	.9	—
	Good grade:																	
	Total edible:																	
302	Raw (75% lean, 25% fat)	57.6	293	17.6	24.1	0	0	.8	10	161	2.7			50	.08	.16	4.2	—
303	Cooked, broiled (67% lean, 33% fat)	45.7	365	24.1	29.1	0	0	1.1	11	198	3.1			50	.07	.19	4.9	—
	Separable lean:																	
304	Raw	72.6	135	21.7	4.7	0	0	1.0	13	202	3.3			10	.09	.19	5.2	—
305	Cooked, broiled	61.0	190	31.5	6.1	0	0	1.4	13	249	3.8			10	.08	.24	6.1	—
	Separable fat:																	
306	Raw	13.8	751	5.3	80.7	0	0	.2	3	43	.8			160	.02	.05	1.3	—
	Hipbone sirloin steak:																	
	Choice grade:																	
	Total edible:																	
307	Raw (61% lean, 39% fat)	46.0	412	14.5	38.8	0	0	.7	8	132	2.2			80	.06	.13	3.5	—
308	Cooked, broiled (55% lean, 45% fat)	35.1	487	19.1	44.9	0	0	.9	9	163	2.5			80	.06	.16	4.0	—
	Separable lean:																	
309	Raw	68.2	179	20.9	9.9	0	0	1.0	12	194	3.1			20	.09	.19	5.0	—
310	Cooked, broiled	56.3	240	29.8	12.5	0	0	1.4	12	239	3.6			20	.08	.23	5.8	—
	Separable fat:																	
311	Raw	12.0	771	4.5	83.3	0	0	.2	3	36	.7			170	.02	.04	1.1	—
	Good grade:																	
	Total edible:																	
312	Raw (64% lean, 36% fat)	50.4	367	15.7	33.2	0	0	.7	9	143	2.3			70	.07	.14	3.8	—
313	Cooked, broiled (58% lean, 42% fat)	39.0	441	21.0	39.0	0	0	1.0	9	176	2.7			70	.06	.17	4.4	—

[30] Average value for 100 grams, all cuts, is 65 mg. for raw beef and 60 mg. for cooked beef. See also Notes on Foods, p. 179.

[31] Average value per 100 grams of beef of all cuts is 355 mg. for raw meat and 370 mg. for cooked meat.

TABLE 1.—COMPOSITION OF FOODS, 100 GRAMS, EDIBLE PORTION—Continued

[Numbers in parentheses denote values imputed—usually from another form of the food or from a similar food. Zero in parentheses indicates that the amount of a constituent probably is none or is too small to measure. Dashes denote lack of reliable data for a constituent believed to be present in measurable amount. Calculated values, as those based on a recipe, are not in parentheses]

Item No.	Food and description	Water	Food energy	Protein	Fat	Carbohydrate: Total	Carbohydrate: Fiber	Ash	Calcium	Phosphorus	Iron	Sodium	Potassium	Vitamin A value	Thiamine	Riboflavin	Niacin	Ascorbic acid
(A)	(B)	(C)	(D)	(E)	(F)	(G)	(H)	(I)	(J)	(K)	(L)	(M)	(N)	(O)	(P)	(Q)	(R)	(S)
		Percent	Calories	Grams	Grams	Grams	Grams	Grams	Milligrams	Milligrams	Milligrams	Milligrams	Milligrams	International units	Milligrams	Milligrams	Milligrams	Milligrams
	Beef[4]—Continued																	
	Retail cuts, trimmed to retail level—Continued																	
	Loin end or sirloin—Continued																	
	Hipbone sirloin steak—Continued																	
	Good grade—Continued																	
	Separable lean:																	
314	Raw	70.9	152	21.4	6.7	0	0	1.0	12	199	3.2			10	0.09	0.19	5.1	—
315	Cooked, broiled	59.2	209	30.8	8.6	0	0	1.4	12	245	3.7			10	.08	.23	6.0	—
	Separable fat:																	
316	Raw	14.4	744	5.5	79.9	0	0	.2	3	45	.8			160	.03	.05	1.3	—
	Short plate:																	
	Choice grade:																	
	Total edible:																	
317	Raw (59% lean, 41% fat)	47.2	400	14.8	37.3	0	0	.7	8	135	2.2			70	.06	.13	3.6	—
318	Cooked, simmered (58% lean, 42% fat)	36.0	474	20.6	42.8	0	0	.6	9	101	2.7			80	.04	.16	3.2	—
	Separable lean:																	
319	Raw	69.7	164	21.1	8.2	0	0	1.0	12	196	3.2			20	.09	.19	5.1	—
320	Cooked, simmered	59.1	222	29.7	10.5	0	0	.8	13	146	3.8			20	.05	.22	4.5	—
	Separable fat:																	
321	Raw	15.3	734	5.9	78.6	0	0	.2	3	49	.9			160	.03	.05	1.4	—
	Good grade:																	
	Total edible:																	
322	Raw (62% lean, 38% fat)	51.3	356	16.1	31.9	0	0	.7	9	147	2.4			60	.07	.14	3.8	—
323	Cooked, simmered (61% lean, 39% fat)	39.9	432	22.3	37.3	0	0	.6	9	110	2.9			70	.04	.17	3.4	—
	Separable lean:																	
324	Raw	71.5	146	21.5	6.0	0	0	1.0	12	200	3.2			10	.09	.19	5.2	—
325	Cooked, simmered	61.1	199	30.3	7.7	0	0	.8	13	149	3.8			10	.05	.23	4.6	—
	Separable fat:																	
326	Raw	18.2	701	7.2	74.3	0	0	.3	4	62	1.1			150	.03	.06	1.7	—
	Rib:																	
	Entire rib, (6th–12th ribs):																	
	Choice grade:																	
	Total edible:																	
327	Raw (64% lean, 36% fat)	47.2	401	14.8	37.4	0	0	.6	9	151	2.2			70	.06	.13	3.6	—
328	Cooked, roasted (64% lean, 36% fat)	40.0	440	19.9	39.4	0	0	.7	9	186	2.6	(20)	(21)	80	.05	.15	3.6	—
	Separable lean:																	
329	Raw	66.8	193	20.7	11.6	0	0	.9	12	208	3.1			20	.09	.18	5.0	—
330	Cooked, roasted	57.2	241	28.2	13.4	0	0	1.1	12	256	3.6			20	.07	.21	5.1	—
	Separable fat:																	
331	Raw	12.8	762	4.8	82.2	0	0	.2	3	54	.7			160	.02	.04	1.2	—
	Ribs, 11th–12th:																	
	Choice grade:																	
	Total edible:																	
332	Raw (55% lean, 45% fat)	43.0	444	13.7	42.7	0	0	.6	8	124	2.1			90	.06	.12	3.3	—
333	Cooked, roasted (55% lean, 45% fat)	36.3	481	18.3	44.7	0	0	.7	8	153	2.4			90	.05	.14	3.4	—
	Separable lean:																	
334	Raw	66.9	192	20.7	11.5	0	0	.9	12	192	3.1			20	.09	.18	5.0	—
335	Cooked, roasted	57.3	240	28.2	13.3	0	0	1.1	12	237	3.6			20	.07	.21	5.1	—
	Separable fat:																	
336	Raw	13.3	756	5.0	81.5	0	0	.2	3	41	.8			160	.02	.04	1.2	—
	Good grade:																	
	Total edible:																	
337	Raw (63% lean, 37% fat)	[illegible].5	376	15.5	34.3	0	0	.7	9	142	2.3			70	.07	.14	3.7	—
338	Cooked, roasted (63% lean, 37% fat)	41.9	417	20.9	36.3	0	0	.9	9	175	2.7			70	.06	.16	3.8	—
	Separable lean:																	
339	Raw	69.5	166	21.1	8.4	0	0	1.0	12	196	3.2			20	.09	.19	5.1	—
340	Cooked, roasted	59.7	215	28.9	10.2	0	0	1.3	12	242	3.7			20	.07	.22	5.2	—
	Separable fat:																	
341	Raw	16.0	726	6.2	77.6	0	0	.2	4	52	.9			160	.03	.06	1.5	—
	Rib, 6th or blade:																	
	Choice grade:																	
	Total edible:																	
342	Raw (71% lean, 29% fat)	50.7	363	16.0	32.7	0	0	.7	9	146	2.4			70	.07	.14	3.8	—
343	Cooked, braised (70% lean, 30% fat)	39.3	437	22.1	38.0	0	0	.6	10	109	2.9			70	.04	.17	3.4	—

	Separable lean:																	
344	Raw	66.1	200	20.5	12.5	0	0	.9	12	190	3.1			20	.09	.18	4.9	—
345	Cooked, braised	55.1	263	28.5	15.7	0	0	.7	13	142	3.7			30	.05	.22	4.4	—
	Separable fat:																	
346	Raw	12.6	764	4.7	82.5	0	0	.2	3	38	.7			160	.02	.04	1.1	—
	Good grade:																	
	Total edible:																	
347	Raw (77% lean, 23% fat)	56.6	300	17.5	25.0	0	0	.8	10	162	2.6			50	.08	.16	4.2	—
348	Cooked, braised (76% lean, 24% fat)	45.1	373	24.3	29.9	0	0	.7	10	121	3.2			60	.05	.19	3.8	—
	Separable lean:																	
349	Raw	69.3	168	21.1	8.6	0	0	1.0	12	196	3.2			20	.09	.19	5.1	—
350	Cooked, braised	58.6	225	29.6	10.9	0	0	.8	13	146	3.8			20	.05	.22	4.5	—
	Separable fat:																	
351	Raw	14.7	741	5.6	79.5	0	0	.2	3	46	.8			160	.02	.05	1.3	—
	Round, entire (round and heel of round):																	
	Choice grade:																	
	Total edible:																	
352	Raw (89% lean, 11% fat)	66.6	197	20.2	12.3	0	0	.9	12	203	3.0			20	.09	.18	4.8	—
353	Cooked, broiled (81% lean, 19% fat)	54.7	261	28.6	15.4	0	0	1.3	12	250	3.5			30	.08	.22	5.6	—
	Separable lean:																	
354	Raw	72.7	135	21.6	4.7	0	0	1.0	13	217	3.2			10	.09	.19	5.2	—
355	Cooked, broiled	61.2	189	31.3	6.1	0	0	1.4	13	268	3.7	[20]	[21]	10	.08	.24	6.0	—
	Separable fat:																	
356	Raw	18.7	696	7.5	73.6	0	0	.2	4	80	1.1			150	.03	.07	1.8	—
	Rump:																	
	Choice grade:																	
	Total edible:																	
357	Raw (75% lean, 25% fat)	56.5	303	17.4	25.3	0	0	.8	10	160	2.6			50	.08	.16	4.2	—
358	Cooked, roasted (75% lean, 25% fat)	48.1	347	23.6	27.3	0	0	1.0	10	197	3.1			50	.06	.18	4.3	—
	Separable lean:																	
359	Raw	70.3	158	21.2	7.5	0	0	1.0	12	197	3.2			20	.09	.19	5.1	—
360	Cooked, roasted	60.4	208	29.1	9.3	0	0	1.3	12	243	3.7			20	.07	.22	5.2	—
	Separable fat:																	
361	Raw	16.0	726	6.2	77.6	0	0	.2	4	52	.9			160	.03	.06	1.5	—
	Good grade:																	
	Total edible:																	
362	Raw (76% lean, 24% fat)	59.4	271	18.3	21.4	0	0	.8	11	168	2.7			40	.08	.16	4.4	—
363	Cooked, roasted (76% lean, 24% fat)	50.7	317	24.9	25.4	0	0	1.0	11	207	3.1			40	.06	.19	4.5	—
	Separable lean:																	
364	Raw	72.0	141	21.6	5.4	0	0	1.0	13	201	3.2			10	.09	.19	5.2	—
365	Cooked, roasted	62.0	190	29.6	7.1	0	0	1.3	13	248	3.7			10	.08	.22	5.3	—
	Separable fat:																	
366	Raw	19.0	692	7.5	73.2	0	0	.3	4	65	1.1			150	03	.07	1.8	—
	Hamburger (ground beef):																	
	Lean:																	
367	Raw	68.3	179	20.7	10.0	0	0	1.0	12	192	3.1	—	—	20	.09	.18	5.0	—
368	Cooked	60.0	219	27.4	11.3	0	0	1.3	12	230	3.5	48	558	20	.09	.23	6.0	—
	Regular ground:																	
369	Raw	60.2	268	17.9	21.2	0	0	.7	10	156	2.7	—	236	40	.08	.16	4.3	—
370	Cooked	54.2	286	24.2	20.3	0	0	1.3	11	194	3.2	47	450	40	.09	.21	5.4	—
	Beef and vegetable stew:																	
371	Cooked (home recipe, with lean beef chuck)	82.4	89	6.4	4.3	6.2	.4	.7	12	75	1.2	37	250	980	.06	.07	1.9	7
372	Canned	82.5	79	5.8	3.1	7.1	.3	1.5	12	45	.9	411	174	970	.03	.05	1.0	3
373	**Beef, canned, roast beef**	60.	224	25.	13.	0	0	2.	16	116	2.4	—	259	—	.02	.23	4.2	0
	Beef, corned, boneless:																	
374	Uncooked, medium-fat	54.2	293	15.8	25.	0	0	5.0	9	125	2.4	1,300	60	—	.03	.15	1.7	0
375	Cooked, medium-fat	43.9	372	22.9	30.4	0	0	2.9	9	93	2.9	1,740	150	—	.02	.18	1.5	0
	Canned:																	
376	Fat	55.3	263	23.5	18.	0	0	3.2	19	98	4.0	—	—	—	.01	.22	3.2	0
377	Medium-fat	59.3	216	25.3	12.	0	0	3.4	20	106	4.3	—	—	—	.02	.24	3.4	0
378	Lean	62.0	185	26.4	8.	0	0	3.6	21	110	4.5	—	—	—	.02	.25	3.5	0
379	Canned corned-beef hash (with potato)	67.4	181	8.8	11.3	10.7	.5	1.8	13	67	2.0	540	200	—	.01	.09	2.1	—
	Beef, dried, chipped:																	
380	Uncooked	47.7	203	34.3	6.3	0	0	11.6	20	404	5.1	4,300	200	—	(.07)	(.32)	(3.8)	0
381	Cooked, creamed	72.0	154	8.2	10.3	7.1	Trace	2.4	105	140	.8	716	153	360	.06	.19	.6	Trace
	Beef, potted. See Sausage, cold cuts, and luncheon meats: item 2008.																	
	Beef potpie:																	
382	Home-prepared, baked	55.1	246	10.1	14.5	18.8	.4	1.5	14	71	1.8	284	159	820	.11	.12	2.0	3
383	Commercial, frozen, unheated	63.3	192	7.3	9.9	18.0	.1	1.5	10	48	1.0	366	93	410	.03	.06	1.2	Trace
	Beer. See Beverages, item 394.																	
	Beets, common, red:																	
384	Raw	87.3	43	1.6	.1	9.9	.8	1.1	16	33	.7	60	335	20	.03	.05	.4	10
385	Cooked, boiled, drained	90.9	32	1.1	.1	7.2	.8	.7	14	23	.5	43	208	20	.03	.04	.3	6

[20] Average value for 100 grams, all cuts, is 65 mg. for raw beef and 60 mg. for cooked beef. See also Notes on Foods, p. 179.

[21] Average value per 100 grams of beef of all cuts is 355 mg. for raw meat and 370 mg. for cooked meat.

TABLE 1.—COMPOSITION OF FOODS, 100 GRAMS, EDIBLE PORTION—Continued

[Numbers in parentheses denote values imputed—usually from another form of the food or from a similar food. Zero in parentheses indicates that the amount of a constituent probably is none or is too small to measure. Dashes denote lack of reliable data for a constituent believed to be present in measurable amount. Calculated values, as those based on a recipe, are not in parentheses]

Item No.	Food and description	Water	Food energy	Protein	Fat	Carbohydrate		Ash	Calcium	Phosphorus	Iron	Sodium	Potassium	Vitamin A value	Thiamine	Riboflavin	Niacin	Ascorbic acid
						Total	Fiber											
(A)	(B)	(C)	(D)	(E)	(F)	(G)	(H)	(I)	(J)	(K)	(L)	(M)	(N)	(O)	(P)	(Q)	(R)	(S)
	Beets, common, red—Continued	Percent	Calories	Grams	Grams	Grams	Grams	Grams	Milligrams	Milligrams	Milligrams	Milligrams	Milligrams	International units	Milligrams	Milligrams	Milligrams	Milligrams
	Canned:																	
	Regular pack:																	
386	Solids and liquid	90.3	34	0.9	0.1	7.9	0.5	0.8	14	17	0.6	[9] 236	167	10	0.01	0.02	0.1	3
387	Drained solids	89.3	37	1.0	.1	8.8	.8	.8	19	18	.7	[9] 236	167	20	.01	.03	.1	3
388	Drained liquid	92.2	26	.8	Trace	6.2	Trace	.8	5	15	.4	[9] 236	167	Trace	.01	.02	.1	3
	Special dietary pack (low-sodium):																	
389	Solids and liquid	90.8	32	.9	Trace	7.8	.5	.5	14	17	.6	46	167	10	.01	.02	.1	3
390	Drained solids	89.8	37	.9	.1	8.7	.8	.5	19	18	.7	46	167	20	.01	.03	.1	3
391	Drained liquid	92.8	25	.8	Trace	5.9	Trace	.5	5	15	.4	46	167	Trace	.01	.02	.1	3
	Beet greens, common:																	
392	Raw	90.9	24	2.2	.3	4.6	1.3	2.0	119	40	3.3	130	570	6,100	.10	.22	.4	30
393	Cooked, boiled, drained	93.6	18	1.7	.2	3.3	1.1	1.2	99	25	1.9	76	332	5,100	.07	.15	.3	15
	Beverages, alcoholic and carbonated nonalcoholic:																	
	Alcoholic:																	
394	Beer, alcohol 4.5% by volume (3.6% by weight)	92.1	[22] 42	.3	0	3.8	—	.2	5	30	Trace	7	25	—	Trace	.03	.6	—
	Gin, rum, vodka, whisky:																	
395	80-proof (33.4% alcohol by weight)	66.6	[22] 231	—	—	Trace	—	—	—	—	—	1	2	—	—	—	—	—
396	86-proof (36.0% alcohol by weight)	64.0	[22] 249	—	—	Trace	—	—	—	—	—	1	2	—	—	—	—	—
397	90-proof (37.9% alcohol by weight)	62.1	[22] 263	—	—	Trace	—	—	—	—	—	1	2	—	—	—	—	—
398	94-proof (39.7% alcohol by weight)	60.3	[22] 275	—	—	Trace	—	—	—	—	—	1	2	—	—	—	—	—
399	100-proof (42.5% alcohol by weight)	57.5	[22] 295	—	—	Trace	—	—	—	—	—	1	2	—	—	—	—	—
	Wines:[4]																	
400	Dessert, alcohol 18.8% by volume (15.3% by weight).	76.7	[22] 137	.1	0	7.7	—	.2	8	—	—	4	75	—	.01	.02	.2	—
401	Table, alcohol 12.2% by volume (9.9% by weight).	85.6	[22] 85	.1	0	4.2	—	.2	9	10	.4	5	92	—	Trace	.01	.1	—
	Carbonated, nonalcoholic:																	
	Carbonated waters:																	
402	Sweetened (quinine sodas)	92.	31	(0)	(0)	8.	(0)	—	—	—	—	—	—	(0)	(0)	(0)	(0)	(0)
403	Unsweetened (club sodas)	100.	0	(0)	(0)	0.	(0)	—	—	—	—	—	—	(0)	(0)	(0)	(0)	(0)
404	Cola type	90.	39	(0)	(0)	10.	(0)	—	—	—	—	—	—	(0)	(0)	(0)	(0)	(0)
405	Cream sodas	89.	43	(0)	(0)	11.	(0)	—	—	—	—	—	—	(0)	(0)	(0)	(0)	(0)
406	Fruit-flavored sodas (citrus, cherry, grape, strawberry, Tom Collins mixer, other) (10%–13% sugar).	88.	46	(0)	(0)	12.	(0)	—	—	—	—	—	—	(0)	(0)	(0)	(0)	(0)
407	Ginger ale, pale dry and golden	92.	31	(0)	(0)	8.	(0)	—	—	—	—	—	—	(0)	(0)	(0)	(0)	(0)
408	Root beer	89.5	41	(0)	(0)	10.5	(0)	—	—	—	—	—	—	(0)	(0)	(0)	(0)	(0)
409	Special dietary drinks with artificial sweetener (less than 1 Calorie per ounce).	100.	—	(0)	(0)	—	(0)	—	—	—	—	—	—	(0)	(0)	(0)	(0)	(0)
	Biscuits, baking powder, baked from home recipe, made with—																	
410	Enriched flour [23]	27.4	369	7.4	17.0	45.8	.2	2.4	121	175	1.6	626	117	Trace	.21	.21	1.8	Trace
411	Unenriched flour [23]	27.4	369	7.4	17.0	45.8	.2	2.4	121	175	.5	626	117	Trace	.04	.10	.5	Trace
412	Self-rising flour, enriched	26.8	372	7.1	17.4	46.0	.2	2.7	[24] 209	[24] 317	1.7	[24] 660	64	Trace	.22	.22	2.1	Trace
	Biscuit dough, commercial, with enriched flour:																	
413	Chilled in cans	37.5	277	7.3	6.4	46.4	.2	2.4	53	497	1.7	868	65	Trace	.26	.17	2.1	0
414	Frozen	30.9	327	5.7	11.9	48.9	.1	2.6	71	400	1.4	910	86	Trace	.22	.17	1.7	Trace
	Biscuit mix, with enriched flour, and biscuits baked from mix:																	
415	Mix, dry form	7.5	424	7.7	12.6	68.7	.3	3.5	27	265	[25] 3.1	1,300	80	Trace	[25] .44	[25] .26	[25] 3.0	Trace
416	Biscuits, made with milk	28.5	325	7.1	9.3	52.3	.2	2.8	68	232	[26] 2.3	973	116	Trace	[26] .27	[26] .25	[26] 2.0	Trace
417	**Blackberries,** including dewberries, boysenberries and youngberries, raw.	84.5	58	1.2	.9	12.9	4.1	.5	32	19	.9	1	170	200	.03	.04	.4	21
	Blackberries, canned, solids and liquid:																	
418	Water pack, with or without artificial sweetener	89.3	40	.8	.6	9.0	2.8	.3	22	13	.6	1	115	140	.02	.02	.2	7
419	Juice pack	85.8	54	.8	.8	12.1	2.7	.5	25	17	.9	1	170	150	.02	.03	.3	10
	Sirup pack:																	
420	Light	81.0	72	.8	.6	17.3	2.7	.3	21	12	.6	1	111	130	.01	.02	.2	7
421	Heavy	76.1	91	.8	.6	22.2	2.6	.3	21	12	.6	1	109	130	.01	.02	.2	7
422	Extra heavy	71.2	110	.8	.6	27.1	2.6	.3	20	12	.6	1	107	130	.01	.02	.2	7
	Blackberries, frozen. See Boysenberries, items 436–437.																	
423	**Blackberry juice,** canned, unsweetened	90.9	37	.3	.6	7.8	Trace	.4	12	12	(.9)	(1)	(170)	—	(.02)	(.03)	(.3)	(10)
	Blackeye peas. See Cowpeas, items 896–904.																	

	Blackfish. See Tautog, item 2275.																	
	Blanc mange. See Puddings, item 1824.																	
	Blueberries:																	
424	Raw	83.2	62	.7	.5	15.3	1.5	.3	15	13	1.0	1	81	100	(.03)	(.06)	(.5)	14
	Canned, solids and liquid:																	
425	Water pack, with or without artificial sweetener	89.3	39	.5	.2	9.8	1.0	.2	10	9	.7	1	60	40	.01	.01	.2	7
426	Sirup pack, extra heavy	73.2	101	.4	.2	26.0	.9	.2	9	8	.6	1	55	40	.01	.01	.2	6
	Frozen, not thawed:																	
427	Unsweetened	85.0	55	.7	.5	13.6	1.5	.2	10	13	.8	1	81	70	.03	.06	.5	7
428	Sweetened	72.3	105	.6	.3	26.5	.9	.3	6	11	.4	1	66	30	.04	.05	.4	8
	Bluefish:																	
429	Raw	75.4	117	20.5	3.3	0	0	1.2	23	243	.6	74	—	—	.12	.09	1.9	—
	Cooked:																	
430	Baked or broiled [27]	68.0	159	26.2	5.2	0	0	1.4	29	287	.7	104	—	50	.11	.10	1.9	—
431	Fried [28]	60.8	205	22.7	9.8	4.7	—	2.0	35	257	.9	146	—	—	.11	.11	1.8	—
	Bockwurst. See Sausage, cold cuts, and luncheon meats: item 1981.																	
	Bologna. See Sausage, cold cuts, and luncheon meats: items 1982–1985.																	
432	**Bonito,** including Atlantic, Pacific, and striped; raw	67.6	168	24.0	7.3	0	0	1.4	—	—	—	—	—	—	—	—	—	—
433	**Boston brown bread**	45.0	211	5.5	1.3	45.6	.7	2.6	90	160	1.9	251	292	[29]0	.11	.06	1.2	0
434	**Bouillon** cubes or powder	4.	120	20.	3.	5.	—	68.	—	—	—	24,000	100	—	—	—	—	—
	Boysenberries:																	
435	Canned, water pack, solids and liquid, with or without artificial sweetener.	89.8	36	.7	.1	9.1	1.9	.3	(19)	(19)	(1.2)	1	85	130	(.01)	(.10)	(.7)	7
	Frozen, not thawed:																	
436	Unsweetened	86.8	48	1.2	.3	11.4	2.7	.3	25	24	1.6	1	153	(170)	.02	.13	1.0	13
437	Sweetened	74.3	96	.8	.3	24.4	1.8	.2	17	17	.6	1	105	(140)	.02	.10	.6	8
438	**Brains,** all kinds (beef, calf, hog, sheep), raw	78.9	125	10.4	8.6	.8	0	1.4	10	312	2.4	125	219	0	.23	.26	4.4	18
	Bran:																	
439	Added sugar and malt extract	3.6	240	12.6	3.0	74.3	7.8	6.5	70	1,176	([30])	1,060	1,070	(0)	[31].10	.29	17.8	Trace
440	Added sugar and defatted wheat germ	3.0	238	10.8	1.8	78.8	6.5	5.6	73	977	8.8	490	—	(0)	.28	.21	14.0	(0)
441	**Bran flakes** (40% bran), added thiamine	3.0	303	10.2	1.8	80.6	3.6	4.4	71	495	4.4	925	—	(0)	.40	.17	6.2	(0)
442	**Bran flakes with raisins,** added thiamine	7.3	287	8.3	1.4	79.3	3.0	3.7	56	396	4.0	800	—	Trace	.32	.13	5.3	(0)
	Braunschweiger. See Sausage, cold cuts, and luncheon meats: item 1986.																	
443	**Brazilnuts**	4.6	654	14.3	66.9	10.9	3.1	3.3	186	693	3.4	1	715	Trace	.96	.12	1.6	—
	Breads: [32]																	
444	Cracked-wheat	34.9	263	8.7	2.2	52.1	.5	2.1	88	128	1.1	529	134	Trace	.12	.09	1.3	Trace
445	Toasted	22.5	313	10.4	2.6	62.0	.6	2.5	105	152	1.3	630	160	Trace	.11	.11	1.5	Trace
	French or vienna:																	
446	Enriched	30.6	290	9.1	3.0	55.4	.2	1.9	43	85	2.2	580	90	Trace	.28	.22	2.5	Trace
447	Toasted	19.3	338	10.6	3.5	64.4	.2	2.2	50	99	2.6	674	105	Trace	.26	.25	2.9	Trace
448	Unenriched	30.6	290	9.1	3.0	55.4	.2	1.9	43	85	.7	580	90	Trace	.08	.08	.8	Trace
449	Toasted	19.3	338	10.6	3.5	64.4	.2	2.2	50	99	.8	674	105	Trace	.08	.10	.9	Trace
	Italian:																	
450	Enriched	31.8	276	9.1	.8	56.4	.2	1.9	17	77	2.2	585	74	(0)	.29	.20	2.6	(0)
451	Unenriched	31.8	276	9.1	.8	56.4	.2	1.9	17	77	.7	585	74	(0)	.09	.06	.8	(0)
452	Raisin	35.3	262	6.6	2.8	53.6	.9	1.7	71	87	1.3	365	233	Trace	.05	.09	.7	Trace
453	Toasted	22.0	316	8.0	3.4	64.6	1.1	2.0	86	105	1.6	440	281	Trace	.05	.11	.8	Trace
	Rye:																	
454	American (⅓ rye, ⅔ clear flour)	35.5	243	9.1	1.1	52.1	.4	2.2	75	147	1.6	557	145	(0)	.18	.07	1.4	(0)
455	Toasted	25.0	282	10.6	1.3	60.5	.5	2.6	87	171	1.9	648	169	(0)	.17	.08	1.6	(0)
456	Pumpernickel	34.0	246	9.1	1.2	53.1	1.1	2.6	84	229	2.4	569	454	(0)	.23	.14	1.2	(0)
457	Salt-rising	36.5	267	7.9	2.4	52.2	.2	1.0	23	69	.6	265	67	10	.04	.05	.6	Trace
458	Toasted	29.4	297	8.8	2.7	58.0	.2	1.1	26	77	.7	294	74	10	.04	.05	.6	Trace
	White:																	
	Enriched, made with—																	
459	1%–2% nonfat dry milk	35.8	269	8.7	3.2	50.4	.2	1.9	70	87	2.4	507	85	Trace	.25	.17	2.3	Trace
460	Toasted	25.3	314	10.1	3.7	58.7	.2	2.2	81	101	2.8	590	99	Trace	.23	.20	2.7	Trace
461	3%–4% nonfat dry milk [33]	35.6	270	8.7	3.2	50.5	.2	2.0	84	97	2.5	507	105	Trace	.25	.21	2.4	Trace
462	Toasted	25.1	314	10.1	3.7	58.8	.2	2.3	98	113	2.9	590	122	Trace	.23	.24	2.8	Trace
463	5%–6% nonfat dry milk	35.0	275	9.0	3.8	50.2	.2	2.0	96	102	2.5	495	121	Trace	.27	.20	2.4	Trace
464	Toasted	24.4	320	10.5	4.4	58.4	.2	2.3	112	119	2.9	576	141	Trace	.25	.23	2.8	Trace

[4] See Notes on Foods, p. 181.

[9] Estimated average based on addition of salt in the amount of 0.6 percent of the finished product.

[22] See Notes on Foods, p. 181, concerning calculation of energy values.

[23] Values are based on biscuits made with baking powder, item 130, and cooking fats, item 999.

[24] Based on use of self-rising flour, item 2445, containing anhydrous monocalcium phosphate. With flour containing leavening ingredients noted in footnote 169, approximate values per 100 grams are: Calcium, 124 mg.; phosphorus, 363 mg.; sodium, 826 mg.

[25] With unenriched flour, approximate values per 100 grams are: Iron, 0.6 mg.; thiamine, 0.05 mg.; riboflavin, 0.05 mg.; niacin, 0.7 mg.

[26] With unenriched flour, approximate values per 100 grams are: Iron, 0.5 mg.; thiamine, 0.04 mg.; riboflavin, 0.10 mg.; niacin, 0.5 mg.

[27] Prepared with butter or margarine.

[28] Prepared with egg, milk or water, and bread crumbs.

[29] Applies to product made with white cornmeal. With yellow degermed cornmeal, value is 70 I.U. per 100 grams.

[30] Values range from 4 to 12 mg. per 100 grams.

[31] For product containing added thiamine, value is 0.4 mg. per 100 grams.

[32] For additional data and information, see discussion of bread and rolls in Notes on Foods, p. 172.

[33] When amount of nonfat dry milk in commercial bread is unknown, values for bread with 3 to 4 percent nonfat dry milk, item 461 or item 467, are suggested. See also Notes on Foods, p. 172.

TABLE 1.—COMPOSITION OF FOODS, 100 GRAMS, EDIBLE PORTION—Continued

[Numbers in parentheses denote values imputed—usually from another form of the food or from a similar food. Zero in parentheses indicates that the amount of a constituent probably is none or is too small to measure. Dashes denote lack of reliable data for a constituent believed to be present in measurable amount. Calculated values, as those based on a recipe, are not in parentheses]

Item No.	Food and description	Water	Food energy	Protein	Fat	Carbohydrate		Ash	Calcium	Phosphorus	Iron	Sodium	Potassium	Vitamin A value	Thiamine	Riboflavin	Niacin	Ascorbic acid
						Total	Fiber											
(A)	(B)	(C)	(D)	(E)	(F)	(G)	(H)	(I)	(J)	(K)	(L)	(M)	(N)	(O)	(P)	(Q)	(R)	(S)
		Percent	*Calories*	*Grams*	*Grams*	*Grams*	*Grams*	*Grams*	*Milligrams*	*Milligrams*	*Milligrams*	*Milligrams*	*Milligrams*	*International units*	*Milligrams*	*Milligrams*	*Milligrams*	*Milligrams*
	Breads [32]—Continued																	
	White—Continued																	
	Unenriched, made with—																	
465	1%-2% nonfat dry milk	35.8	269	8.7	3.2	50.4	0.2	1.9	70	87	0.7	507	85	Trace	0.09	0.08	1.2	Trace
466	Toasted	25.3	314	10.1	3.7	58.7	.2	2.2	81	101	.8	590	99	Trace	.08	.09	1.4	Trace
467	3%-4% nonfat dry milk [33]	35.6	270	8.7	3.2	50.5	.2	2.0	84	97	.7	507	105	Trace	.07	.09	1.1	Trace
468	Toasted	25.1	314	10.1	3.7	58.8	.2	2.3	98	113	.8	590	122	Trace	.06	.10	1.3	Trace
469	5%-6% nonfat dry milk	35.0	275	9.0	3.8	50.2	.2	2.0	96	102	.7	495	121	Trace	.07	.13	.9	Trace
470	Toasted	24.4	320	10.5	4.4	58.4	.2	2.3	112	119	.8	576	141	Trace	.07	.15	1.0	Trace
	Whole-wheat, made with—																	
471	2% nonfat dry milk	36.4	243	10.5	3.0	47.7	1.6	2.4	99	228	2.3	527	273	Trace	.26	.12	2.8	Trace
472	Toasted	24.3	289	12.5	3.6	56.7	1.9	2.9	118	271	2.7	627	325	Trace	.25	.15	3.4	Trace
473	Water	36.4	241	9.1	2.6	49.3	1.5	2.6	84	254	2.3	530	256	Trace	.30	.10	2.8	Trace
474	Toasted	24.3	287	10.8	3.1	58.7	1.8	3.1	100	302	2.7	631	305	Trace	.29	.12	3.3	Trace
	See also Biscuits; Boston brown bread; Cornbread; Muffins; Rolls; Salt sticks.																	
475	**Breadcrumbs**, dry, grated	6.5	392	12.6	4.6	73.4	.3	2.9	122	141	3.6	736	152	Trace	.22	.30	3.5	Trace
476	**Bread pudding** with raisins	58.6	187	5.6	6.1	28.4	.1	1.3	109	114	1.1	201	215	300	.06	.19	.1	1
	Bread sticks (vienna). See Salt sticks, item 1966.																	
	Bread stuffing mix and stuffings prepared from mix:																	
477	Mix, dry form	6.3	371	12.9	3.8	72.4	.8	4.6	124	189	3.2	1,331	172	Trace	.22	.26	3.2	Trace
	Stuffing:																	
478	Dry, crumbly: prepared with water, table fat	33.2	358	6.5	21.8	35.6	.4	2.9	66	97	1.6	896	90	650	.09	.12	1.5	Trace
479	Moist: prepared with water, egg, table fat	61.4	208	4.4	12.8	19.7	.2	1.7	40	66	1.0	504	58	420	.05	.09	.8	Trace
480	**Breadfruit**, raw	70.8	103	1.7	.3	26.2	1.2	1.0	33	32	1.2	15	439	40	.11	.03	.9	29
	Breakfast cereals. See Corn, Oats, Rice, Wheat, also Bran, Farina.																	
	Broadbeans, raw:																	
481	Immature seeds	72.3	105	8.4	.4	17.8	2.2	1.1	27	157	2.2	4	471	220	.28	.17	1.6	30
482	Mature seeds, dry	11.9	338	25.1	1.7	58.2	6.7	3.1	102	391	7.1	—	—	70	.50	.30	2.5	—
	Broccoli:																	
483	Raw spears	89.1	32	3.6	.3	5.9	1.5	1.1	103	78	1.1	15	382	[34]2,500	.10	.23	.9	113
484	Cooked spears, boiled, drained	91.3	26	3.1	.3	4.5	1.5	.8	88	62	.8	10	267	2,500	.09	.20	.8	90
	Frozen:																	
	Chopped:																	
485	Not thawed	90.6	29	3.2	.3	5.2	1.1	.7	58	59	.7	17	241	2,600	.07	.13	.6	70
486	Cooked, boiled, drained	91.6	26	2.9	.3	4.6	1.1	.6	54	56	.7	15	212	2,600	.06	.12	.5	57
	Spears:																	
487	Not thawed	90.7	28	3.3	.2	5.1	1.1	.7	43	60	.7	13	244	1,900	.07	.13	.6	78
488	Cooked, boiled, drained	91.4	26	3.1	.2	4.7	1.1	.6	41	58	.7	12	220	1,900	.06	.11	.5	73
	Brown betty. See Apple brown betty, item 25.																	
	Brownies. See Cookies, items 813-814.																	
	Brussels sprouts:																	
489	Raw	85.2	45	4.9	.4	8.3	1.6	1.2	36	80	1.5	14	390	550	.10	.16	.9	102
490	Cooked, boiled, drained	88.2	36	4.2	.4	6.4	1.6	.8	32	72	1.1	10	273	520	.08	.14	.8	87
	Frozen:																	
491	Not thawed	88.4	36	3.3	.2	7.3	1.2	.8	22	62	.9	16	328	570	.10	.11	.6	87
492	Cooked, boiled, drained	89.3	33	3.2	.2	6.5	1.2	.8	21	61	.8	14	295	570	.08	.10	.6	81
	Buckwheat:																	
493	Whole-grain	11.0	335	11.7	2.4	72.9	9.9	2.0	114	282	3.1	—	448	(0)	.60	—	4.4	(0)
	Flour:																	
494	Dark	12.	333	11.7	2.5	72.0	1.6	1.8	33	347	2.8	—	—	(0)	.58	.15	2.9	(0)
495	Light	12.	347	6.4	1.2	79.5	.5	.9	11	88	1.0	—	320	(0)	.08	(.04)	(.4)	(0)
	Buckwheat pancake mix. See Pancake mix, item 1461.																	
496	**Buffalofish**, raw	77.4	113	17.5	4.2	0	0	1.1	—	—	—	52	293	—	—	—	—	—
	Bulgur (parboiled wheat):																	
	Dry, commercial, made from—																	
497	Club wheat	9.	359	8.7	1.4	79.5	1.7	1.4	30	319	4.7	—	262	(0)	.30	.10	4.2	(0)
498	Hard red winter wheat	10.	354	11.2	1.5	75.7	1.7	1.6	29	338	3.7	—	229	(0)	.28	.14	4.5	(0)
499	White wheat	(9.)	357	10.3	1.2	78.1	1.3	1.4	36	300	(4.7)	—	310	(0)	(.30)	(.10)	(4.2)	(0)
	Canned, made from hard red winter wheat:																	
500	Unseasoned [35]	56.0	168	6.2	.7	35.0	.8	2.1	20	200	1.3	599	87	(0)	.05	.03	2.4	(0)
501	Seasoned [36]	56.0	182	6.2	3.3	32.8	.8	1.7	20	195	1.4	460	112	(0)	.06	.04	3.0	(0)
502	**Bullhead, black**, raw	81.3	84	16.3	1.6	0	0	1.0	—	—	—	—	—	—	—	—	—	—

	Bullocksheart. See Custardapple, item 949.																	
	Burbot:																	
503	Raw	81.1	82	17.4	.9	0	0	1.0	—	190	—	—	—	—	.39	.14	1.5	—
504	Cooked, fried	60.5	—	37.0	—	0	0	—	—	—	—	—	—	—	.54	.23	3.7	—
	Burghul. See Bulgur, items 497–501.																	
505	**Butter** [37]	15.5	716	.6	81.	.4	0	2.5	20	16	0	987	23	3,300	—	—	—	0
506	**Butter oil or dehydrated butter**	.2	876	.3	99.5	0	0	0	—	—	—	—	—	4,080	—	—	—	0
	Butterfish, raw:																	
507	From northern waters	71.4	169	18.1	10.2	0	0	1.4	—	—	—	—	—	—	—	—	—	—
508	From gulf waters	78.2	95	16.2	2.9	0	0	2.9	—	—	—	—	—	—	—	—	—	—
	Buttermilk:																	
509	Fluid, cultured (made from skim milk)	90.5	36	3.6	.1	5.1	0	.7	121	95	Trace	130	140	Trace	.04	.18	.1	1
510	Dried	2.8	387	34.3	5.3	50.0	0	7.6	1,248	970	.6	507	1,606	220	.26	1.72	.9	—
511	**Butternuts**	3.8	629	23.7	61.2	8.4	—	2.9	—	—	6.8	—	—	—	—	—	—	—
	Cabbage:																	
	Common varieties (Danish, domestic, and pointed types):																	
512	Raw	92.4	24	1.3	.2	5.4	.8	.7	49	29	.4	20	233	130	.05	.05	.3	[38]47
	Cooked, boiled until tender, drained:																	
513	Shredded, cooked in small amount of water	93.9	20	1.1	.2	4.3	.8	.5	44	20	.3	14	163	130	.04	.04	.3	33
514	Wedges, cooked in large amount of water	94.3	18	1.0	.2	4.0	.8	.5	42	17	.3	13	151	120	.02	.02	.1	24
515	Dehydrated	4.	308	12.4	1.7	73.7	10.3	8.2	405	287	3.9	190	2,207	1,300	[39].45	.40	3.0	[39]211
516	Red, raw	90.2	31	2.0	.2	6.9	1.0	.7	42	35	.8	26	268	40	.09	.06	.4	61
517	Savoy, raw	92.0	24	2.4	.2	4.6	.8	.8	67	54	.9	22	269	200	.05	.08	.3	55
518	**Cabbage, Chinese** (also called celery cabbage or petsai), compact heading type, raw.	95.0	14	1.2	.1	3.0	.6	.7	43	40	.6	23	253	150	.05	.04	.6	25
	Cabbage, spoon (also called white mustard cabbage or pakchoy), nonheading green leaf type:																	
519	Raw	94.3	16	1.6	.2	2.9	.6	1.0	165	44	.8	26	306	3,100	.05	.10	.8	25
520	Cooked, boiled, drained	95.2	14	1.4	.2	2.4	.6	.8	148	33	.6	18	214	3,100	.04	.08	.7	15
	Cabbage salad. See Coleslaw, items 801–804.																	
	Cakes:																	
	Baked from home recipes: [40]																	
521	Angelfood	31.5	269	7.1	.2	60.2	0	1.0	9	22	.2	283	88	0	.01	.14	.2	0
522	Boston cream pie	34.5	302	5.0	9.4	49.9	0	1.2	67	101	.5	186	89	210	.03	.11	.2	Trace
	Caramel:																	
523	Without icing	23.0	385	4.5	17.3	53.7	.1	1.5	78	106	1.3	305	68	180	.02	.08	.2	Trace
524	With caramel icing	20.9	379	3.7	14.8	59.1	0	1.5	84	95	1.5	252	64	200	.02	.07	.1	Trace
	Chocolate (devil's food):																	
525	Without icing	24.6	366	4.8	17.2	52.0	.3	1.4	74	137	.9	294	140	150	.02	.10	.2	Trace
526	With chocolate icing	22.0	369	4.5	16.4	55.8	.3	1.3	70	131	1.0	235	154	160	.02	.10	.2	Trace
527	With uncooked white icing	21.3	369	3.8	14.6	59.2	.2	1.1	59	106	.7	234	110	180	.02	.08	.2	Trace
	Cottage pudding, made with enriched flour:																	
528	Without sauce	26.6	344	6.4	11.3	54.3	.1	1.4	90	115	1.4	299	88	140	.15	.17	1.2	Trace
529	With chocolate sauce	27.9	318	5.3	8.8	56.7	.3	1.3	71	109	1.4	233	140	100	.12	.14	1.0	Trace
530	With fruit sauce (strawberry)	36.6	292	5.1	8.8	48.4	.3	1.1	73	93	1.2	233	93	120	.12	.15	1.1	12
	Fruitcake, made with enriched flour:																	
531	Dark	18.1	379	4.8	15.3	59.7	.6	2.1	72	113	2.6	158	496	120	.13	.14	.8	Trace
532	Light	18.7	389	6.0	16.5	57.4	.7	1.4	68	115	1.6	193	233	70	.10	.11	.7	Trace
533	Gingerbread, made with enriched flour	30.8	317	3.8	10.7	52.0	.1	2.7	68	65	2.3	237	454	90	.12	.11	.9	0
	Plain cake or cupcake:																	
534	Without icing	24.5	364	4.5	13.9	55.9	.1	1.2	64	102	.4	300	79	170	.02	.09	.2	Trace
535	With chocolate icing	21.4	368	4.2	13.9	59.4	.2	1.1	63	104	.6	229	114	180	.02	.09	.2	Trace
536	With boiled white icing	22.9	352	3.8	10.5	61.8	Trace	1.0	49	77	.3	262	64	130	.02	.07	.2	Trace
537	With uncooked white icing	20.6	367	3.4	11.8	63.3	Trace	.9	50	75	.3	227	61	200	.02	.07	.1	Trace
	Pound:																	
538	Old-fashioned (equal weights flour, sugar, table fat, eggs).	17.2	473	5.7	29.5	47.0	.1	.6	21	79	.8	110	60	280	.03	.09	.2	0
539	Modified	19.4	411	6.4	18.7	54.7	.1	.9	40	104	.8	178	78	290	.04	.11	.2	Trace
540	Sponge	31.8	297	7.6	5.7	54.1	0	.8	30	112	1.2	167	87	450	.05	.14	.2	Trace
	White:																	
541	Without icing	24.2	375	4.6	16.0	54.0	.1	1.2	63	91	.2	323	76	30	.01	.08	.2	Trace
542	With coconut icing	21.3	371	3.7	13.3	60.7	.3	1.0	45	72	.3	257	106	20	.01	.07	.2	Trace
543	With uncooked white icing	20.0	375	3.3	12.9	62.9	0	.9	48	65	.1	234	58	110	.01	.06	.1	Trace
	Yellow:																	
544	Without icing	23.5	363	4.5	12.7	58.2	.1	1.1	71	112	.4	258	78	150	.02	.08	.2	Trace
545	With caramel icing	21.8	362	4.0	11.7	61.3	.1	1.2	77	163	.7	226	73	170	.02	.08	.2	Trace
546	With chocolate icing	21.2	365	4.2	13.0	60.4	.2	1.1	68	112	.6	208	108	160	.02	.08	.2	Trace
	Frozen, commercial, devil's food:																	
547	With chocolate icing	21.0	380	4.3	17.6	55.6	.3	1.5	54	92	.8	420	119	430	.02	.08	.2	Trace
548	With whipped-cream filling, chocolate icing	29.7	371	3.5	21.9	43.8	.2	1.1	80	122	.6	190	113	270	.02	.08	.2	Trace

[33] When amount of nonfat dry milk in commercial bread is unknown, values for bread with 3 to 4 percent nonfat dry milk, item 461 or item 467, are suggested. See also Notes on Foods, p. 172.

[34] Value for leaves is 16,000 I.U. per 100 grams; flower clusters, 3,000 I.U.; stalks, 400 I.U.

[35] Processed, partially debranned, whole-kernel wheat with salt added.

[36] Processed, partially debranned, whole-kernel wheat with chicken fat, chicken stock base, dehydrated onion flakes, salt, monosodium glutamate, and herbs.

[37] Values apply to salted butter. Unsalted butter contains less than 10 mg. of either sodium or potassium per 100 grams. Value for vitamin A is the year-round average.

[38] For freshly harvested cabbage, average value is 51 mg. per 100 grams; for stored cabbage, 42 mg. per 100 grams.

[39] Applies to unsulfited product. For sulfited product, values per 100 grams are: Thiamine, 0.10 mg.; ascorbic acid, 300 mg.

[40] Unenriched cake flour used unless otherwise specified. Values for cakes that contain baking powder and/or fat are based on use of baking powder, item 130, and cooking fats, item 999. See also Notes on Foods, p. 173.

TABLE 1.—COMPOSITION OF FOODS, 100 GRAMS, EDIBLE PORTION—Continued

[Numbers in parentheses denote values imputed—usually from another form of the food or from a similar food. Zero in parentheses indicates that the amount of a constituent probably is none or is too small to measure. Dashes denote lack of reliable data for a constituent believed to be present in measurable amount. Calculated values, as those based on a recipe, are not in parentheses]

Item No.	Food and description	Water	Food energy	Protein	Fat	Carbohydrate		Ash	Calcium	Phosphorus	Iron	Sodium	Potassium	Vitamin A value	Thiamine	Riboflavin	Niacin	Ascorbic acid
						Total	Fiber											
(A)	(B)	(C)	(D)	(E)	(F)	(G)	(H)	(I)	(J)	(K)	(L)	(M)	(N)	(O)	(P)	(Q)	(R)	(S)
	Cake mixes and cakes baked from mixes:	*Percent*	*Calories*	*Grams*	*Grams*	*Grams*	*Grams*	*Grams*	*Milligrams*	*Milligrams*	*Milligrams*	*Milligrams*	*Milligrams*	*International units*	*Milligrams*	*Milligrams*	*Milligrams*	*Milligrams*
	Angelfood:																	
549	Mix, dry form	1.8	385	8.4	0.2	88.5	Trace	1.1	108	125	0.4	190	112	0	0.01	0.17	0.2	0
550	Cake, made with water, flavorings	34.0	259	5.7	.2	59.4	Trace	.7	95	119	.3	146	60	0	Trace	.11	.1	0
	Chocolate malt:																	
551	Mix, dry form	3.8	412	4.0	10.7	79.0	0.2	2.5	100	270	1.0	551	119	70	.04	.08	.4	0
552	Cake, made with eggs, water, uncooked white icing.	19.8	346	3.4	8.7	66.6	.1	1.5	63	166	.7	318	80	190	.03	.07	.2	Trace
	Coffeecake, with enriched flour:																	
553	Mix, dry form	3.8	431	5.9	11.0	77.2	.2	2.1	36	191	[a]2.0	613	87	Trace	[a].30	[a].14	[a]2.4	Trace
554	Cake, made with egg, milk	30.0	322	6.3	9.6	52.4	.1	1.7	61	174	[a]1.6	431	109	160	[a].18	[a].16	[a]1.4	Trace
	Cupcake:																	
555	Mix, dry form	4.9	438	3.7	13.6	75.8	.3	2.0	173	263	.4	596	46	0	.05	.06	.3	0
556	Cake, made with eggs, milk, without icing	25.6	350	4.9	12.0	55.8	.2	1.7	161	235	.5	453	84	150	.04	.11	.2	Trace
557	Cake, made with eggs, milk, chocolate icing	22.2	358	4.5	12.6	59.2	.3	1.5	130	197	.8	335	117	170	.04	.11	.2	Trace
	Devil's food:																	
558	Mix, dry form	3.9	406	4.8	11.7	77.0	.3	2.6	80	120	1.2	457	121	Trace	.03	.08	.5	Trace
559	Cake, made with eggs, water, chocolate icing	23.6	339	4.4	12.3	58.3	.3	1.4	59	105	.8	262	130	150	.03	.08	.3	Trace
	Gingerbread:																	
560	Mix, dry form	3.0	425	5.4	10.4	78.2	.1	3.0	180	200	1.4	463	418	Trace	.04	.14	.4	Trace
561	Cake, made with water	37.0	276	3.1	6.8	51.1	Trace	2.0	90	100	1.6	304	274	Trace	.03	.09	.8	Trace
	Honey spice:																	
562	Mix, dry form	3.5	443	4.3	14.0	76.3	.4	1.9	74	274	.2	373	99	Trace	.02	.08	.3	Trace
563	Cake, made with eggs, water, caramel icing	22.7	352	4.1	10.8	60.9	.2	1.5	71	193	.8	245	82	160	.02	.09	.2	Trace
	Marble:																	
564	Mix, dry form	4.0	425	4.9	13.5	75.6	.1	2.0	130	270	1.0	381	188	Trace	.03	.09	.4	Trace
565	Cake, made with eggs, water, boiled white icing	23.6	331	4.4	8.7	62.0	.1	1.3	78	171	.8	259	122	90	.02	.08	.2	Trace
	White:																	
566	Mix, dry form	3.4	434	4.1	11.9	78.4	.2	2.2	150	270	.2	373	88	Trace	.02	.07	.3	Trace
567	Cake, made with egg whites, water, chocolate icing.	21.1	351	3.9	10.7	62.8	.2	1.5	99	179	.5	227	116	60	.02	.08	.2	Trace
	Yellow:																	
568	Mix, dry form	3.3	438	4.0	12.9	77.6	.1	2.2	140	270	.2	407	86	Trace	.02	.07	.3	Trace
569	Cake, made with eggs, water, chocolate icing	25.6	337	4.1	11.3	57.6	.2	1.4	91	182	.6	227	109	140	.02	.08	.2	Trace
	Cake icings:																	
570	Caramel	14.1	360	1.3	6.7	76.5	0	1.4	102	63	2.0	83	52	280	.01	.06	Trace	Trace
571	Chocolate	14.3	376	3.2	13.9	67.4	.4	.9	60	111	1.2	61	195	210	.02	.10	.2	Trace
572	Coconut	15.0	364	1.9	7.7	74.9	.8	.5	6	30	.5	118	167	0	.01	.04	.2	0
	White:																	
573	Uncooked	11.1	376	.5	6.6	81.6	0	.2	15	12	Trace	49	18	270	Trace	.02	Trace	Trace
574	Boiled	17.9	316	1.4	0	80.3	0	.4	2	2	Trace	143	18	0	Trace	.03	Trace	0
	Cake icing mixes and icings made from mixes:																	
	Chocolate fudge:																	
575	Mix, dry form	.8	409	2.5	9.8	86.4	.6	.5	18	82	1.3	95	78	Trace	.01	.06	.3	0
576	Icing, made with water, table fat	15.3	378	2.2	14.4	67.0	.5	1.1	16	66	1.0	156	63	270	.01	.04	.2	0
	Creamy fudge (contains nonfat dry milk):																	
577	Mix, dry form	3.1	386	3.2	7.4	85.1	.6	1.2	45	102	1.3	265	111	Trace	.02	.09	.3	Trace
	Icing:																	
578	Made with water	15.1	339	2.8	6.5	74.6	.5	1.0	39	89	1.1	232	97	Trace	.02	.08	.3	Trace
579	Made with water, table fat	15.1	383	2.6	15.2	65.9	.5	1.2	37	81	1.0	321	89	390	.02	.07	.3	Trace
	Candied fruits. See Apricots, Cherries, Citron, Figs, Ginger root, Grapefruit peel, Lemon peel, Orange peel, Pear, Pineapple.																	
	Candy:																	
580	Butterscotch	1.5	397	Trace	3.4	94.8	0	.3	17	6	1.4	66	2	140	0	Trace	Trace	0
	Candy corn. See Fondant, item 602.																	
	Caramels:																	
581	Plain or chocolate	7.6	399	4.0	10.2	76.6	.2	1.5	148	122	1.4	226	192	10	.03	.17	.2	Trace
582	Plain or chocolate, with nuts	7.1	428	4.5	16.3	70.5	.4	1.6	140	139	1.5	203	233	20	.11	.17	.2	Trace
583	Chocolate-flavored roll	5.6	396	2.2	8.2	82.7	.2	1.2	68	119	1.8	197	123	Trace	.02	.07	.1	Trace
	Chocolate:																	
584	Bittersweet	1.8	477	7.9	39.7	46.8	1.8	2.3	58	284	5.0	3	615	40	.03	.17	1.0	0
585	Semisweet	1.1	507	4.2	35.7	57.0	1.0	1.2	30	150	2.6	2	325	20	.01	.08	.5	0
586	Sweet	.9	528	4.4	35.1	57.9	.5	1.2	94	142	1.4	33	269	19	.02	.14	.3	Trace

	Chocolate, milk:																	
587	Plain	.9	520	7.7	32.3	56.9	.4	1.9	228	231	1.1	94	384	270	.06	.34	.3	Trace
588	With almonds	1.5	532	9.3	35.6	51.3	.7	2.0	229	272	1.6	80	442	230	.08	.41	.8	Trace
589	With peanuts	1.0	543	14.1	38.1	44.6	.9	2.0	174	294	1.4	66	487	180	.25	.26	5.0	Trace
	Chocolate-coated:																	
590	Almonds	2.0	569	12.3	43.7	39.6	1.5	2.3	203	343	2.8	59	546	Trace	.12	.53	1.7	Trace
591	Chocolate fudge	6.2	430	3.8	16.0	73.1	.2	.9	101	110	1.3	228	193	Trace	.04	.13	.2	0
592	Chocolate fudge, with nuts	6.0	452	4.9	20.8	67.3	.4	1.0	101	137	1.5	205	219	Trace	.06	.13	.2	Trace
593	Coconut center	6.6	438	2.8	17.6	72.0	.6	1.0	48	77	1.1	197	165	0	.02	.07	.2	0
594	Fondant	5.8	410	1.7	10.5	81.0	.1	.9	57	54	1.1	185	91	Trace	.03	.06	.1	Trace
595	Fudge, caramel, and peanuts	8.3	433	7.7	18.1	64.1	.4	1.7	179	186	1.4	204	301	Trace	.16	.22	1.9	Trace
596	Fudge, peanuts, and caramel	7.0	459	9.4	23.1	58.7	.7	1.7	127	192	1.1	128	222	Trace	.26	.15	3.7	Trace
597	Honeycombed hard candy, with peanut butter	1.7	463	6.6	19.5	70.6	.4	1.5	80	135	1.8	163	225	Trace	.05	.09	2.9	Trace
598	Nougat and caramel	7.7	416	4.0	13.9	72.8	.2	1.4	127	123	1.6	173	211	40	.06	.17	.2	Trace
599	Peanuts	1.0	561	16.4	41.3	39.1	1.2	2.0	116	298	1.5	60	504	Trace	.37	.18	7.4	Trace
600	Raisins	4.8	425	5.4	17.1	70.5	.6	2.1	152	174	2.5	64	603	150	.08	.21	.4	Trace
601	Vanilla creams	7.5	435	3.8	17.1	70.3	.1	1.2	128	110	.6	182	178	Trace	.05	.07	.1	Trace
602	Fondant	7.6	364	.1	2.0	89.6	Trace	.7	14	6	1.1	212	5	0	Trace	Trace	Trace	0
	Fudge:																	
603	Chocolate	8.2	400	2.7	12.2	75.0	.2	1.8	77	84	1.0	190	147	Trace	.02	.09	.2	Trace
604	Chocolate, with nuts	7.8	426	3.9	17.4	69.0	.4	1.8	79	114	1.2	171	177	Trace	.04	.09	.3	Trace
605	Vanilla	10.0	398	3.0	11.1	74.8	0	1.1	112	83	.5	208	127	Trace	.02	.13	.1	Trace
606	Vanilla, with nuts	9.4	424	4.2	16.4	68.8	.2	1.2	111	113	.8	187	114	Trace	.05	.13	.1	Trace
607	Gum drops, starch jelly pieces	11.7	347	.1	.7	87.4	0	.1	6	Trace	.5	35	5	0	0	Trace	Trace	0
608	Hard	1.4	386	0	1.1	97.2	0	.3	21	7	1.9	32	4	0	0	0	0	0
609	Jelly beans	6.3	367	Trace	.5	93.1	Trace	.1	12	4	1.1	12	1	0	0	Trace	Trace	0
610	Marshmallows	17.3	319	2.0	Trace	80.4	0	.3	18	6	1.6	39	6	0	0	Trace	Trace	0
	Mints, uncoated. See Fondant, item 602.																	
611	Peanut bars	1.5	515	17.5	32.2	47.2	1.2	1.6	44	273	1.8	10	448	0	.43	.08	9.4	0
612	Peanut brittle (no added salt or soda)	2.0	421	5.7	10.4	81.0	.5	.9	35	95	2.3	31	151	0	.16	.03	3.4	0
	Sugar-coated:																	
613	Almonds	2.3	456	7.8	18.6	70.2	.9	1.1	100	166	1.9	20	255	0	.05	.27	1.0	0
614	Chocolate discs	1.2	466	5.2	19.7	72.7	.3	1.2	135	140	1.3	72	250	100	.06	.20	.3	Trace
	Cantaloups. See Muskmelons, item 1358.																	
	Cape-gooseberries. See Groundcherries, item 1092.																	
	Capicola. See Sausage, cold cuts, and luncheon meats: item 1989.																	
615	**Carambola, raw**	90.4	35	.7	.5	8.0	.9	.4	4	17	1.5	2	192	1,200	.04	.02	.3	35
	Caribou. See Reindeer, items 1855–1858.																	
616	**Carissa (natalplum) raw**	80.8	70	.5	1.3	16.0	.9	.4	—	—	—	—	—	40	.04	.06	.2	38
617	**Carob flour (St. Johnsbread)**	11.2	180	4.5	1.4	80.7	7.7	2.2	352	81	—	—	—	—	—	—	—	—
618	**Carp, raw**	77.8	115	18.0	4.2	0	0	1.1	50	253	.9	50	286	170	.01	.04	1.5	1
	Carrots:																	
619	Raw	88.2	42	1.1	.2	9.7	1.0	.8	37	36	.7	47	341	[43] 11,000	.06	.05	.6	8
620	Cooked, boiled, drained	91.2	31	.9	.2	7.1	1.0	.6	33	31	.6	33	222	10,500	.05	.05	.5	6
	Canned:																	
	Regular pack:																	
621	Solids and liquid	91.8	28	.6	.2	6.5	.6	.9	25	20	.7	[9] 236	120	10,000	.02	.02	.4	2
622	Drained solids	91.2	30	.8	.3	6.7	.8	1.0	30	22	.7	[9] 236	120	15,000	.02	.03	.4	2
623	Drained liquid	93.3	22	.4	0	5.5	Trace	.8	14	15	.8	[9] 236	120	Trace	.02	.02	.4	2
	Special dietary pack (low-sodium):																	
624	Solids and liquid	93.7	22	.7	.1	5.0	.6	.5	25	20	.7	39	120	10,000	.02	.02	.4	2
625	Drained solids	93.0	25	.8	.1	5.6	.8	.5	30	22	.7	39	120	15,000	.02	.03	.4	2
626	Drained liquid	95.2	16	.4	0	4.0	Trace	.4	14	15	.8	39	120	Trace	.02	.02	.4	2
627	Dehydrated	4.	341	6.6	1.3	81.1	9.3	7.0	256	234	6.0	268	1,944	100,000	.31	.30	3.0	15
	Casaba melon. See Muskmelons, item 1359.																	
628	**Cashew nuts**	5.2	561	17.2	45.7	29.3	1.4	2.6	38	373	3.8	[44] 15	464	100	.43	.25	1.8	—
629	**Catfish, freshwater, raw**	78.0	103	17.6	3.1	0	0	1.3	—	—	.4	60	330	—	.04	.03	1.7	—
	Catsup. See Tomato catsup, item 2286.																	
	Cauliflower:																	
630	Raw	91.0	27	2.7	.2	5.2	1.0	.9	25	56	1.1	13	295	60	.11	.10	.7	78
631	Cooked, boiled, drained	92.8	22	2.3	.2	4.1	1.0	.6	21	42	.7	9	206	60	.09	.08	.6	55
	Frozen:																	
632	Not thawed	92.9	22	2.0	.2	4.3	.8	.6	19	42	.6	11	225	30	.06	.06	.5	56
633	Cooked, boiled, drained	94.0	18	1.9	.2	3.3	.8	.6	17	38	.5	10	207	30	.04	.05	.4	41
	Caviar, sturgeon:																	
634	Granular	46.0	262	26.9	15.0	3.3	—	8.8	276	355	11.8	2,200	180	—	—	—	—	—
635	Pressed	36.0	316	34.4	16.7	4.9	—	8.0	—	—	—	—	—	—	—	—	—	—
636	**Celeriac, root, raw**	88.4	40	1.8	.3	8.5	1.3	1.0	43	115	.6	100	300	—	.05	.06	.7	8
	Celery, all, including green and yellow varieties:																	
637	Raw	94.1	17	.9	.1	3.9	.6	1.0	39	28	.3	126	341	[45] 240	.03	.03	.3	9
638	Cooked, boiled, drained	95.3	14	.8	.1	3.1	.6	.7	31	22	.2	88	239	230	.02	.03	.3	6
	Cereals, breakfast. See Corn, Oats, Rice, Wheat, also Bran, Farina.																	

[9] Estimated average based on addition of salt in the amount of 0.6 percent of the finished product.

[41] With unenriched flour, approximate values per 100 grams are: Iron, 0.5 mg.; thiamine, 0.07 mg.; riboflavin, 0.06 mg.; niacin, 1.0 mg.

[42] With unenriched flour, approximate values per 100 grams are: Iron, 0.6 mg.; thiamine, 0.05 mg.; riboflavin, 0.11 mg.; niacin, 0.6 mg.

[43] Average for carrots marketed as fresh vegetable. See also Notes on Foods, p. 175.

[44] Applies to unsalted nuts. For salted nuts, value is approximately 200 mg. per 100 grams.

[45] Average for all varieties. For green varieties, value is 270 I.U. per 100 grams; for yellow varieties, 140 I.U.

TABLE 1.—COMPOSITION OF FOODS, 100 GRAMS, EDIBLE PORTION—Continued

[Numbers in parentheses denote values imputed—usually from another form of the food or from a similar food. Zero in parentheses indicates that the amount of a constituent probably is none or is too small to measure. Dashes denote lack of reliable data for a constituent believed to be present in measurable amount. Calculated values, as those based on a recipe, are not in parentheses]

Item No.	Food and description	Water	Food energy	Protein	Fat	Carbohydrate		Ash	Calcium	Phosphorus	Iron	Sodium	Potassium	Vitamin A value	Thiamine	Riboflavin	Niacin	Ascorbic acid
						Total	Fiber											
(A)	(B)	(C)	(D)	(E)	(F)	(G)	(H)	(I)	(J)	(K)	(L)	(M)	(N)	(O)	(P)	(Q)	(R)	(S)
	Cervelat. See Sausage, cold cuts, and luncheon meats: items 1990–1991.	*Percent*	*Calories*	*Grams*	*Grams*	*Grams*	*Grams*	*Grams*	*Milligrams*	*Milligrams*	*Milligrams*	*Milligrams*	*Milligrams*	*International units*	*Milligrams*	*Milligrams*	*Milligrams*	*Milligrams*
	Chard, Swiss:																	
639	Raw	91.1	25	2.4	0.3	4.6	0.8	1.6	88	39	3.2	147	550	6,500	0.06	0.17	0.5	32
640	Cooked, boiled, drained	93.7	18	1.8	.2	3.3	.7	1.0	73	24	1.8	86	321	5,400	.04	.11	.4	16
641	**Charlotte russe,** with ladyfingers, whipped-cream filling.	45.5	286	5.9	14.6	33.5	Trace	.5	46	91	.7	43	64	740	.03	.10	.1	Trace
642	**Chayote,** raw	91.8	28	.6	.1	7.1	.7	.4	13	26	.5	5	102	20	.03	.03	4	19
	Cheeses, natural and processed; cheese foods; cheese spreads:																	
	Natural cheeses:																	
643	Blue or Roquefort type	40.	368	21.5	30.5	2.0	0	6.0	315	339	(.5)	—	—	(1,240)	.03	.61	1.2	(0)
644	Brick	41.0	370	22.2	30.5	1.9	0	4.4	730	455	(.9)	—	—	(1,240)	—	.45	.1	(0)
645	Camembert (domestic)	52.2	299	17.5	24.7	1.8	0	3.8	105	184	.5	—	111	(1,010)	.04	.75	.8	(0)
646	Cheddar (domestic type, commonly called American).	37.	398	25.0	32.2	2.1	0	3.7	750	478	1.0	700	82	(1,310)	.03	.46	.1	(0)
	Cottage (large or small curd):																	
647	Creamed	78.3	106	13.6	4.2	2.9	0	1.0	94	152	.3	229	85	(170)	.03	.25	.1	(0)
648	Uncreamed	79.0	86	17.0	.3	2.7	0	1.0	90	175	.4	290	72	(10)	.03	.28	(.1)	(0)
649	Cream	51.	374	8.0	37.7	2.1	0	1.2	62	95	.2	250	74	(1,540)	(.02)	.24	.1	(0)
650	Limburger	45.	345	21.2	28.0	2.2	0	3.6	590	393	.6	—	—	(1,140)	.08	.50	.2	(0)
651	Parmesan	30.	393	36.0	26.0	2.9	0	5.1	1,140	781	.4	734	149	(1,060)	.02	.73	.2	(0)
652	Swiss (domestic)	39.	370	27.5	28.0	1.7	0	3.8	925	563	.9	710	104	(1,140)	.01	(.40)	(.1)	(0)
	Pasteurized process cheese:																	
653	American	40.	370	23.2	30.0	1.9	0	4.9	697	[46] 771	.9	[46] 1,136	80	(1,220)	.02	.41	Trace	(0)
654	Pimiento (American)	40.	371	23.0	30.2	1.8	Trace	5.0	—	—	—	—	—	—	—	—	—	—
655	Swiss	40.	355	26.4	26.9	1.6	0	5.1	887	[46] 867	(.9)	[46] 1,167	100	(1,100)	(.01)	.40	.1	(0)
656	Pasteurized process cheese food, American	43.2	323	19.8	24.0	7.1	0	5.9	570	[46] 754	(.8)	—	—	(980)	(.02)	.58	.2	(0)
657	Pasteurized process cheese spread, American	48.6	288	16.0	21.4	8.2	0	5.8	565	[46] 875	(.6)	[46] 1,625	240	(870)	.01	.54	.1	(0)
658	**Cheese fondue,** from home recipe	54.2	265	14.8	18.3	10.0	Trace	2.7	317	294	1.2	542	165	880	.06	.34	.2	Trace
659	**Cheese souffle,** from home recipe	65.0	218	9.9	17.1	6.2	Trace	1.8	201	195	1.0	364	121	800	.05	.24	.2	Trace
660	**Cheese straws**	21.7	453	11.2	29.9	34.5	.1	2.7	259	206	.6	721	63	390	.02	.16	.3	0
661	**Cherimoya,** raw	73.5	94	1.3	.4	24.0	2.2	.8	23	40	.5	—	—	10	.10	.11	1.3	9
	Cherries:																	
	Raw:																	
662	Sour, red	83.7	58	1.2	.3	14.3	.2	.5	22	19	.4	2	191	1,000	.05	.06	.4	10
663	Sweet	80.4	70	1.3	.3	17.4	.4	.6	22	19	.4	2	191	110	.05	.06	.4	10
664	Candied	12.0	339	.5	.2	86.7	.5	.6	—	—	—	—	—	—	—	—	—	—
	Canned:																	
	Sour, red, solids and liquid:																	
665	Water pack	88.0	43	.8	.2	10.7	.1	.3	15	13	.3	2	130	680	.03	.02	.2	5
	Sirup pack:																	
666	Light	80.0	74	.8	.2	18.7	.1	.3	14	13	.3	1	126	660	.03	.02	.2	5
667	Heavy	76.0	89	.8	.2	22.7	.1	.3	14	12	.3	1	124	650	.03	.02	.2	5
668	Extra heavy	70.1	112	.8	.2	28.6	.1	.3	14	12	.2	1	121	630	.03	.02	.2	5
	Sweet, solids and liquid:																	
669	Water pack, with or without artificial sweetener	86.6	48	.9	.2	11.9	.3	.4	15	13	.3	1	130	60	.02	.02	.2	3
	Sirup pack:																	
670	Light	82.0	65	.9	.2	16.5	.3	.4	15	13	.3	1	128	60	.02	.02	.2	3
671	Heavy	78.0	81	.9	.2	20.5	.3	.4	15	13	.3	1	126	60	.02	.02	.2	3
672	Extra heavy	73.0	100	.8	.2	25.6	.3	.4	14	12	.3	1	123	50	.02	.02	.2	3
	Frozen, not thawed:																	
	Sour, red:																	
673	Unsweetened	84.9	55	1.0	.4	13.4	.3	.3	13	22	.7	2	188	1,000	.04	.07	.3	5
674	Sweetened	70.6	112	1.0	.4	27.8	.2	.2	12	15	.5	2	130	480	.03	.06	.3	6
675	**Cherries, maraschino,** bottled, solids and liquid	70.0	116	.2	.2	29.4	.3	.2	—	—	—	—	—	—	—	—	—	—
676	**Chervil,** raw	80.7	57	3.4	.9	11.5	—	3.5	—	—	—	—	—	—	—	—	—	9
	Chestnuts:																	
677	Fresh	52.5	194	2.9	1.5	42.1	1.1	1.0	27	88	1.7	6	454	—	.22	.22	.6	—
678	Dried	8.4	377	6.7	4.1	78.6	2.5	2.2	52	162	3.3	12	875	—	.32	.38	1.2	—
679	**Chestnut flour**	11.4	362	6.1	3.7	76.2	2.0	2.6	50	164	3.2	11	847	—	.23	.37	1.0	—
680	**Chewing gum**	3.5	317	—	—	95.2	—	1.3	—	—	—	—	—	(0)	(0)	(0)	(0)	(0)

	Chicken:																	
	All classes:																	
	Light meat without skin:																	
681	Raw	73.7	117	23.4	1.9	0	0	1.0	11	218	1.1	50	320	60	.05	.09	10.7	—
682	Cooked, roasted	63.8	166	31.6	3.4	0	0	1.2	11	265	1.3	64	411	60	.04	.10	11.6	—
	Dark meat without skin:																	
683	Raw	73.7	130	20.6	4.7	0	0	1.0	13	188	1.5	67	250	150	.08	.20	5.2	—
684	Cooked, roasted	64.4	176	28.0	6.3	0	0	1.2	13	229	1.7	86	321	150	.07	.23	5.6	—
685	**Broilers,** flesh only, cooked, broiled	71.0	136	23.8	3.8	0	0	1.1	9	201	1.7	66	274	90	.05	.19	8.8	—
	Fryers (weight, ready to cook, with giblets, more than 1¾ lbs.):																	
	Flesh, skin, and giblets:																	
686	Raw	75.7	124	18.6	4.9	0	0	.8	12	201	1.9	—	—	730	.07	.38	5.6	—
687	Cooked, fried	53.3	249	30.7	11.8	2.9	—	1.3	13	254	2.3	—	—	820	.07	.57	9.1	—
	Flesh and skin:																	
688	Raw	75.4	126	18.8	5.1	0	0	.7	11	198	1.5	—	—	170	.05	.23	5.6	—
689	Cooked, fried	53.5	250	30.6	11.9	2.8	—	1.2	12	243	1.8	—	—	170	.06	.36	9.2	—
	Flesh only:																	
690	Raw	77.2	107	19.3	2.7	0	0	.8	12	203	1.3	58	285	90	.06	.25	6.4	—
691	Cooked, fried	58.6	209	31.2	7.8	1.2	—	1.2	13	257	1.6	78	381	90	.06	.35	9.7	—
	Skin only:																	
692	Raw	66.3	223	16.1	17.1	0	0	.5	9	174	2.4	—	—	550	.03	.13	2.0	—
693	Cooked, fried	32.5	419	28.3	28.9	9.1	—	1.2	8	186	2.4	—	—	490	.07	.41	7.0	—
	Giblets:																	
694	Raw	78.4	103	17.5	3.1	.1	0	.9	14	220	4.5	—	—	4,530	.16	1.36	4.9	—
695	Cooked, fried	51.7	252	30.8	11.2	4.7	—	1.6	18	336	6.5	—	—	5,760	.17	2.18	8.0	—
	Light meat with skin:																	
696	Raw	75.4	120	19.9	3.9	0	0	.8	11	211	1.3	—	—	130	.05	.16	6.7	—
697	Cooked, fried	55.0	234	31.5	9.9	2.4	—	1.2	11	260	1.5	—	—	130	.05	.27	11.9	—
	Dark meat with skin:																	
698	Raw	75.3	132	17.7	6.3	0	0	.7	12	185	1.7	—	—	200	.06	.30	4.7	—
699	Cooked, fried	52.1	263	29.9	13.6	3.1	—	1.3	12	228	2.0	—	—	210	.07	.45	6.7	—
	Light meat without skin:																	
700	Raw	77.2	101	20.5	1.5	0	0	.8	11	218	1.1	50	320	50	.05	.17	7.6	—
701	Cooked, fried	59.5	197	32.1	6.1	1.1	—	1.2	12	280	1.3	68	434	50	.05	.25	12.9	—
	Dark meat without skin:																	
702	Raw	77.3	112	18.1	3.8	0	0	.8	13	188	1.5	67	250	120	.06	.34	5.3	—
703	Cooked, fried	57.5	220	30.4	9.3	1.5	—	1.3	14	235	1.8	88	330	130	.07	.45	6.8	—
	Cut-up parts:																	
	Back:																	
704	Raw	73.3	157	16.5	9.6	0	0	.6	12	185	1.7	—	—	310	.05	.23	4.3	—
705	Cooked, fried	40.5	347	30.0	21.2	6.8	0	1.5	15	262	2.7	—	—	390	.07	.50	6.8	—
	Breast:																	
706	Raw	76.0	110	20.8	2.4	0	0	.8	11	214	1.2	—	—	80	.05	.16	7.9	—
707	Cooked, fried	58.4	203	32.5	6.4	1.5	—	1.2	12	276	1.7	—	—	90	.05	.22	14.7	—
	Drumstick:																	
708	Raw	76.5	115	18.8	3.9	0	0	.8	13	186	1.6	—	—	120	.06	.32	4.3	—
709	Cooked, fried	55.0	235	32.6	10.2	1.0	—	1.2	15	236	2.3	—	—	140	.07	.40	7.1	—
	Neck:																	
710	Raw	74.5	151	15.5	9.4	0	0	.6	11	182	1.9	—	—	310	.05	.25	3.0	—
711	Cooked, fried	50.2	289	26.7	17.4	4.5	—	1.2	12	234	2.7	—	—	350	.09	.41	5.7	—
	Rib:																	
712	Raw	76.2	124	17.7	5.4	0	0	.7	11	212	1.3	—	—	170	.04	.18	5.1	—
713	Cooked, fried	45.7	298	31.5	15.4	5.9	—	1.5	13	291	2.0	—	—	210	.05	.47	9.4	—
	Thigh:																	
714	Raw	75.5	128	18.1	5.6	0	0	.8	12	186	1.6	—	—	180	.06	.33	5.7	—
715	Cooked, fried	55.8	237	29.1	11.4	2.5	—	1.2	13	236	2.3	—	—	200	.06	.48	6.8	—
	Wing:																	
716	Raw	73.5	146	18.5	7.4	0	0	.6	10	203	1.5	—	—	240	.04	.14	4.1	—
717	Cooked, fried	52.6	268	29.0	14.8	2.7	—	.9	10	236	2.0	—	—	250	.05	.26	6.8	—
	Roasters:																	
	Total edible:																	
718	Raw	63.0	239	18.2	17.9	0	0	.9	10	176	1.6	—	—	920	.08	.19	6.7	—
719	Cooked, roasted	53.5	290	25.2	20.2	0	0	1.1	10	220	1.9	—	—	960	.07	.22	7.4	—
	Flesh, skin, and giblets:																	
720	Raw	67.5	191	19.6	11.9	0	0	1.0	12	194	1.7	—	—	760	.08	.21	7.3	—
721	Cooked, roasted	57.5	242	27.2	14.0	0	0	1.3	12	242	2.0	—	—	790	.08	.25	8.1	—
	Flesh and skin:																	
722	Raw	66.9	197	19.5	12.6	0	0	1.0	11	191	1.5	—	—	410	.08	.12	7.4	—
723	Cooked, roasted	57.0	248	27.1	14.7	0	0	1.3	11	239	1.8	—	—	420	.08	.14	8.2	—
	Flesh only:																	
724	Raw	73.3	131	21.1	4.5	0	0	1.1	12	203	1.3	58	285	150	.10	.12	7.7	—
725	Cooked, roasted	62.8	183	29.5	6.3	0	0	1.4	12	254	1.5	77	376	150	.10	.15	8.5	—

[46] Values for phosphorus and sodium are based on use of 1.5 percent anhydrous disodium phosphate as the emulsifying agent. If emulsifying agent does not contain either phosphorus or sodium, the content of these two nutrients in milligrams per 100 grams is as follows:

	P	Na
Item 653, American process cheese	444	650
Item 655, Swiss process cheese	540	681
Item 656, American cheese food	427	—
Item 657, American cheese spread	548	1,139

TABLE 1.—COMPOSITION OF FOODS, 100 GRAMS, EDIBLE PORTION—Continued

[Numbers in parentheses denote values imputed—usually from another form of the food or from a similar food. Zero in parentheses indicates that the amount of a constituent probably is none or is too small to measure. Dashes denote lack of reliable data for a constituent believed to be present in measurable amount. Calculated values, as those based on a recipe, are not in parentheses]

Item No.	Food and description	Water	Food energy	Protein	Fat	Carbohydrate		Ash	Calcium	Phosphorus	Iron	Sodium	Potassium	Vitamin A value	Thiamine	Riboflavin	Niacin	Ascorbic acid
						Total	Fiber											
(A)	(B)	(C)	(D)	(E)	(F)	(G)	(H)	(I)	(J)	(K)	(L)	(M)	(N)	(O)	(P)	(Q)	(R)	(S)
		Percent	Calories	Grams	Grams	Grams	Grams	Grams	Milligrams	Milligrams	Milligrams	Milligrams	Milligrams	International units	Milligrams	Milligrams	Milligrams	Milligrams
	Chicken—Continued																	
	Roasters—Continued																	
	Giblets:																	
726	Raw	72.4	135	19.8	4.8	1.7	0	1.3	15	218	4.4	—	—	4,290	0.09	1.07	6.7	6
	Light meat without skin:																	
727	Raw	72.3	128	23.3	3.2	0	0	1.2	11	218	1.1	50	320	100	.08	.08	10.6	—
728	Cooked, roasted	61.3	182	32.3	4.9	0	0	1.5	11	272	1.3	66	422	110	.08	.10	11.8	—
	Dark meat without skin:																	
729	Raw	73.2	132	21.0	4.7	0	0	1.1	13	188	1.5	67	250	150	.13	.16	4.7	—
730	Cooked, roasted	62.7	184	29.3	6.5	0	0	1.4	14	235	1.8	88	330	160	.12	.19	5.3	—
	Hens and cocks:																	
	Total edible:																	
731	Raw	56.9	298	17.4	24.8	0	0	.9	10	167	1.4	—	—	1,080	.06	.19	8.2	—
732	Cooked, stewed	45.9	369	24.0	29.5	0	0	.7	10	123	1.6	—	—	1,190	.04	.21	7.8	—
	Flesh, skin, and giblets:																	
733	Raw	61.7	246	19.0	18.3	0	0	1.0	11	185	1.5	—	—	900	.07	.20	9.1	—
734	Cooked, stewed	50.8	312	26.2	22.2	0	0	.8	11	136	1.8	—	—	990	.04	.23	8.6	—
	Flesh and skin:																	
735	Raw	61.3	251	19.0	18.8	0	0	.9	11	182	1.3	—	—	610	.06	.13	9.2	—
736	Cooked, stewed	50.4	317	26.1	22.8	0	0	.7	11	134	1.5	—	—	670	.04	.14	8.8	—
	Flesh only:																	
737	Raw	70.5	155	21.6	7.0	0	0	1.0	12	203	1.3	58	285	230	.08	.14	10.1	—
738	Cooked, stewed	60.4	208	30.0	8.9	0	0	.8	12	149	1.5	55	272	250	.04	.15	9.6	—
	Giblets:																	
739	Raw	66.8	191	18.6	11.6	1.8	0	1.2	15	214	4.4	—	—	4,300	.09	1.09	6.7	6
	Light meat without skin:																	
740	Raw	71.7	133	23.4	3.7	0	0	1.2	11	218	1.1	50	320	120	.05	.09	11.5	—
741	Cooked, stewed	62.1	180	32.2	4.7	0	0	.9	11	160	1.3	48	306	130	.03	.09	11.0	—
	Dark meat without skin:																	
742	Raw	71.2	154	20.2	7.5	0	0	1.1	13	188	1.5	67	250	240	.10	.18	8.7	—
743	Cooked, stewed	61.1	207	28.5	9.5	0	0	.9	13	138	1.8	64	239	270	.06	.20	8.3	—
	Capons:																	
	Total edible:																	
744	Raw	56.2	283	21.4	21.2	0	0	1.2	—	—	—	—	—	—	—	—	—	—
	Flesh and skin:																	
745	Raw	55.2	291	21.6	22.0	0	0	1.2	—	—	—	—	—	—	—	—	—	—
	Giblets:																	
746	Raw	63.3	220	20.4	14.6	.4	0	1.3	—	—	—	—	—	—	—	—	—	—
747	**Chicken, canned,** meat only, boned	65.2	198	21.7	11.7	0	0	1.4	21	247	1.5	—	138	230	.04	.12	4.4	4
	Chicken, potted. See Sausage, cold cuts, and luncheon meats: item 2008.																	
748	**Chicken a la king,** cooked, from home recipe	68.2	191	11.2	14.0	5.0	Trace	1.6	52	146	1.0	310	165	460	.04	.17	2.2	5
749	**Chicken fricassee,** cooked, from home recipe	71.3	161	15.3	9.3	3.2	Trace	.9	6	113	.9	154	140	70	.02	.07	2.4	0
	Chicken potpie:																	
750	Home-prepared, baked	56.6	235	10.1	13.5	18.3	.4	1.5	30	100	1.3	256	148	1,330	.11	.11	1.8	2
751	Commercial, frozen, unheated	57.8	219	6.7	11.5	22.2	.4	1.8	11	50	1.0	411	153	910	.10	.14	1.4	4
752	**Chicken and noodles,** cooked, from home recipe	71.1	153	9.3	7.7	10.7	Trace	1.2	11	103	.9	250	62	180	.02	.07	1.8	Trace
753	**Chickpeas or garbanzos,** mature seeds, dry, raw	10.7	360	20.5	4.8	61.0	5.0	3.0	150	331	6.9	26	797	50	.31	.15	2.0	—
754	**Chicory, Witloof** (also called French or Belgian endive), bleached head (forced), raw.[47]	95.1	15	1.0	1	3.2	—	.6	18	21	.5	7	182	Trace	—	—	—	—
755	**Chicory greens,** raw	92.8	20	1.8	.3	3.8	.8	1.3	86	40	.9	—	420	4,000	.06	.10	.5	22
	Chili con carne, canned:																	
756	With beans	72.4	133	7.5	6.1	12.2	.6	1.8	32	126	1.7	531	233	60	.03	.07	1.3	—
757	Without beans[48]	66.9	200	10.3	14.8	5.8	.2	2.2	38	152	1.4	—	—	150	.02	.12	2.2	—
	Chili powder. See Peppers, item 1544.																	
	Chili sauce. See Peppers, items 1539, 1542; and Tomatoes, item 2287.																	
758	**Chives,** raw	91.3	28	1.8	.3	5.8	1.1	.8	69	44	1.7	—	250	5,800	.08	.13	.5	56
	Chocolate:																	
759	Bitter or baking[49]	2.3	505	10.7	53.0	28.9	2.5	3.1	78	384	6.7	4	830	60	.05	.24	1.5	0
	Bittersweet. See Candy, item 584.																	
	Chocolate sirup:																	
760	Thin type	31.6	245	2.3	2.0	62.7	.6	1.0	17	92	1.6	52	282	Trace	.02	.07	.4	0
761	Fudge type	25.4	330	5.1	13.7	54.0	.4	1.4	127	159	1.3	89	284	150	.04	.22	.4	Trace

TABLE 4.—CHOLESTEROL CONTENT OF FOODS

[Letters a and b designate items that have the same chemical composition for the edible portion but differ in the amount of refuse. The data in column C apply to 100 grams of edible portion of the item, although it may be purchased with the refuse indicated in column E and described or implied in column B. For information on the nature of the refuse, see comparable items in table 2]

Item No.		Item	Amount of cholesterol in—		Refuse from item as purchased
			100 grams, edible portion	Edible portion of 1 pound as purchased	
(A)		(B)	(C)	(D)	(E)
			Milligrams	*Milligrams*	*Percent*
1		Beef, raw:			
	a	With bone	70	270	15
	b	Without bone	70	320	0
2		Brains, raw	>2,000	>9,000	0
3		Butter	250	1,135	0
4		Caviar or fish roe	>300	>1,300	0
		Cheese:			
5		Cheddar	100	455	0
6		Cottage, creamed	15	70	0
7		Cream	120	545	0
8		Other (25% to 30% fat)	85	385	0
9		Cheese spread	65	295	0
10		Chicken, flesh only, raw	60	------	0
11		Crab:			
	a	In shell	125	270	52
	b	Meat only	125	565	0
12		Egg, whole	550	2,200	12
13		Egg white	0	0	0
		Egg yolk:			
14		Fresh	1,500	6,800	0
15		Frozen	1,280	5,800	0
16		Dried	2,950	13,380	0
17		Fish:			
	a	Steak	70	265	16
	b	Fillet	70	320	0
18		Heart, raw	150	680	0
19		Ice cream	45	205	0
20		Kidney, raw	375	1,700	0
21		Lamb, raw:			
	a	With bone	70	265	16
	b	Without bone	70	320	0
22		Lard and other animal fat	95	430	0
23		Liver, raw	300	1,360	0
24		Lobster:			
	a	Whole	200	235	74
	b	Meat only	200	900	0
		Margarine:			
25		All vegetable fat	0	0	0
26		Two-thirds animal fat, one-third vegetable fat	65	295	0
		Milk:			
27		Fluid, whole	11	50	0
28		Dried, whole	85	385	0
29		Fluid, skim	3	15	0
30		Mutton:			
	a	With bone	65	250	16
	b	Without bone	65	295	0
31		Oysters:			
	a	In shell	>200	>90	90
	b	Meat only	>200	>900	0
32		Pork:			
	a	With bone	70	260	18
	b	Without bone	70	320	0
33		Shrimp:			
	a	In shell	125	390	31
	b	Flesh only	125	565	0
34		Sweetbreads (thymus)	250	1,135	0
35		Veal:			
	a	With bone	90	320	21
	b	Without bone	90	410	0

TABLE 5.—MAGNESIUM CONTENT OF FOODS

[Letters a and b designate items that have the same chemical composition for the edible portion but differ in the amount of refuse. The data in column C apply to 100 grams of edible portion of the item, although it may be purchased with the refuse indicated in column E and described or implied in column B. For information on the nature of the refuse, see comparable items in table 2]

Item No.	Item	Amount of magnesium in— 100 grams, edible portion	Amount of magnesium in— Edible portion of 1 pound as purchased	Refuse from item as purchased
(A)	(B)	(C)	(D)	(E)
		Milligrams	*Milligrams*	*Percent*
1	Almonds, dried:			
a	In shell	270	625	49
b	Shelled	270	1,225	0
	Apples:			
	Raw:			
2	Not pared	8	33	8
3	Pared	5	20	14
	Dried (24% moisture):			
4	Uncooked	22	100	0
5	Cooked, without added sugar	6		
6	Frozen slices, sweetened	4	18	0
7	Apple juice or cider, canned or bottled	4	18	0
8	Applesauce, canned, sweetened	5	23	0
	Apricots:			
9	Raw	12	51	6
10	Canned, solids and liquid	7	32	0
	Dried (25% moisture):			
11	Uncooked	62	281	0
12	Cooked, fruit and liquid, without added sugar	20		
13	Frozen, sweetened	9	41	0
	Asparagus:			
14	Raw	20	51	44
15	Frozen	14	64	0
16	Avocados, all commercial varieties, raw	45	153	25
	Bacon, cured:			
17	Raw:			
a	Sliced	12	54	0
b	Slab	12	51	6
18	Cooked, broiled or fried, drained	25		
	Bacon, Canadian:			
19	Unheated	20	91	0
20	Cooked, broiled or fried, drained	24		
	Bananas:			
21	Raw	33	102	32
22	Dehydrated, or banana powder (3% moisture)	132	599	0
	Barley:			
23	Pearled, light	37	168	0
24	Whole-grain	124	562	0
	Beans, common, mature seeds, dry:			
	White:			
25	Raw	170	771	0
26	Canned, baked	37	168	0
27	Red, raw	163	739	0
	Beans, lima:			
	Immature seeds:			
28	Raw	67	304	0
29	Frozen	48	218	0
30	Mature seeds, dry, raw	180	816	0
	Beans, snap:			
31	Raw	32	128	12
32	Canned, drained solids	14		
33	Frozen	21	95	0

INDEX

D

G

H

I

J